THE
SPIRITUAL
HEART
OF YOUR
HEALTH

D1303566

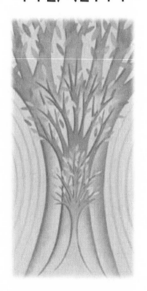

THE SPIRITUAL HEART OF YOUR HEALTH

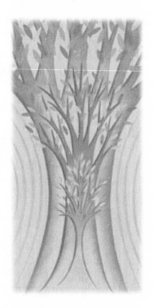

JAMES K. WAGNER

A DEVOTIONAL GUIDE ON THE HEALING STORIES OF JESUS

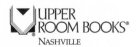

UPPER ROOM BOOKS®
NASHVILLE

The Spiritual Heart of Your Health
A Devotional Guide on the Healing Stories of Jesus

Copyright © 2002 by James K. Wagner
All rights reserved.

No part of this book may be reproduced in any manner whatsoever without written permission of the publisher except in brief quotations embodied in critical articles or reviews. For information, address Upper Room Books®, 1908 Grand Avenue, Nashville, TN 37212.

The Upper Room® Web site: http://www.upperroom.org.

UPPER ROOM®, UPPER ROOM BOOKS® and design logos are trademarks owned by The Upper Room®, Nashville, Tennessee. All rights reserved.

Unless otherwise indicated, scripture quotations in this publication are from the *Contemporary English Version.* © American Bible Society 1991, 1995. Used by permission.

Scripture quotations noted NRSV are from *New Revised Standard Version Bible,* copyright, 1989, Division of Christian Education of the National Council of the Churches of Christ in the United States of America. Used by permission. All rights reserved.

Scripture quotations marked GNT are taken from the Good News Translation—Second Edition; Today's English Version © 1992 American Bible Society.

Scripture quotations marked RSV are from the *Revised Standard Version of the Bible,* copyright, 1952 (2nd edition, 1971) by the Division of Christian Education of the National Council of the Churches of Christ in the United States of America. Used by permission. All rights reserved.

The publisher gratefully acknowledges permission to reproduce copyrighted material appearing in this book. Additional credit lines appear on page 192.

Cover art: Sandra Dionisi/SIS
Cover and interior design: Thelma Whitworth
Interior typesetting: PerfecType
First Printing: 2002

Library of Congress Cataloging-in-Publication Data

Wagner, James K.
    The spiritual heart of your health : a devotional guide on the healing stories of Jesus / by James K. Wagner.
       p. cm.
Includes bibliographical references (p.) and index.
ISBN 0-8358-0958-7
    1. Healing--Religious aspects--Christianity. 2. Spiritual healing--Prayer-books and devotions--English. 3. Healing in the Bible. 4. Jesus Christ--Person and offices. I. Title.

BT732.5 .W34 2002
234'.131--dc21   2001045442

Printed in Canada

To

MARY LOU,

whose spiritual heart

has blessed her husband

and her family

for forty-five years

JESUS SAID,

"I came so that everyone would have life, and have it in its fullest."

JOHN 10:10

THE APOSTLE PAUL WROTE:

"I pray that God, who gives peace, will make you completely holy. And may your spirit, soul, and body be kept healthy and faultless until our Lord Jesus Christ returns."

1 THESSALONIANS 5:23

Spiritual formation is the process whereby we grow in relationship with God and become conformed to Christ.

UPPER ROOM MINISTRIES

CONTENTS

THIRTY SCRIPTURE MEDITATIONS

FOREWORD

You have in your hands a wonderful introduction to the stories of healing that Jesus performed. The Gospel account of these healing experiences is the center of each of these thirty chapters. James K. Wagner has opened the scripture passages that contain these stories as a skilled locksmith opens a vault filled with the treasures of the earth. Not one of the stories is damaged or diminished in its opening. Each story is preserved in its fullness and richness and then is polished just enough with contemporary insight to allow some of its original luster and truth to shine through. Each healing story is prefaced with prayer and completed with benediction in a way that leads the reader into the presence of the Great Physician, where all healing takes place.

All of us need healing. Somewhere along the journey of life we will face the need for healing for ourselves and for those we love. Sometimes that need for healing comes in sudden, catastrophic illness and sometimes in the form of slow, persistent disease that saps our energy and life itself. The need for healing that makes itself known within our own lives is also evident in the lives of those we love. It is never a question of our need for healing; it is only a question of when and where we need God's healing grace to restore us and those we love to wholeness.

In an age of unprecedented scientific discovery about the human body and of unprecedented advances in medicine, we are seeing more clearly than ever the link between spiritual healing and modern medicine. Today the unity of mind, body, and spirit is proclaimed by scientists and theologians alike. *The Spiritual Heart of Your Health* recognizes this unity, welcomes all the best that medical science has to offer, and seeks to introduce the reader to all that faith has to offer for wholeness and wellness. What undergirds both the gift of science and the gift of faith is the loving presence of a God made known in Jesus Christ, a God who desires life abundant for each of us and for whom all things are possible.

Unfortunately Christians do not always claim their full inheritance. We often live as spiritual paupers while we have unlimited resources at our disposal. The treasure house of faith often remains locked, which denies believers access to God's resources. One of those resources is the gift of healing. James Wagner has gleaned thirty healing stories of Jesus and invites the reader to explore each of them in depth. The experience with each story begins in prayer and continues with the author's reflections and the added insight of an authority on the subject of the healing story. The reader then reflects for a time with a series of clearly focused questions before going out into the world abiding in the awareness of God's healing presence.

While the material lends itself to individual use, it is clearly accessible and usable in small groups where the various themes of healing may be explored with others. The devotional treatment of each story makes this resource appropriate for prayer groups, study groups, Sunday school classes, and churchwide studies.

This volume's title reveals the content of the book in a remarkable way. The author's premise is well-founded, well-documented, and clearly stated. We are spiritual beings, and to deny the spiritual nature of our existence is to cut ourselves off from life itself. Life is a spiritual experience, and health is a spiritual gift offered to all who believe in God as made known to us in Jesus Christ. The abundant life that is promised to us is available as we make ourselves available to God. Therefore a major step toward wholeness and health is the establishment of a way of life that keeps us available and open to God's presence and action in our lives. While we need and give thanks for every good gift of modern medicine, we know that wholeness is a larger issue than conquering even the most horrible disease. To be whole and complete and therefore to walk with God in all of life is a spiritual gift that is offered to us in Christ Jesus. But wholeness is a gift we must discover and claim for ourselves. That discovery and claiming is made much easier by the chapters of *The Spiritual Heart of Your Health*.

Will everyone be healed as we anticipate? No, but every Christian may receive the healing gift of grace from God in Christ. And all of us may be more whole and complete than we could ever be without this gift of grace. We can each establish a way of life that is conducive to health and wholeness. This way cooperates with God's desire for life abundant and eternal for each of us. This way of life can keep us in touch with, and open to, God's active grace in our lives. *The Spiritual Heart of Your Health* can help you receive the inheritance that is yours as a child of God. Use this volume prayerfully and slowly as you invite the Great Physician to bring health and wholeness to you and to those you love.

Rueben P. Job
Goodlettsville, Tennessee

PREFACE

More than twenty years ago I wrote *Blessed to Be a Blessing*, basically a how-to book with practical guidelines for starting and maintaining healing ministries in the local church. The genesis of that book emerged in the 1970s with the awakening of the dormant ministry of the Healing Christ by the charismatic renewal movement, the opening of holistic health-care centers, and a revived interest in Bible study, especially study of Jesus' life and ministry.

Continuing research validates and authenticates the significance of paying attention to the spiritual dimensions of life and especially to the spirituality of personal health in the healing process. Dr. David Hilton, former staff member of the Christian Medical Commission of the World Council of Churches, wrote this:

> The most important dimension to health is the spiritual. Even in the midst of poverty some people stay well, while among the world's affluent many are chronically ill. Why? Medical science is beginning to affirm that one's beliefs and feelings are the ultimate tools and powers for healing. Unresolved guilt, anger, resentment, and meaninglessness are found to be the greatest suppressors of the body's powerful, health-controlling immune system, while loving relationships in community are among its strongest augmenters. Those in harmony with the Creator, the earth, and their neighbors not only survive tragedy and suffering best, but grow stronger in the process.[1]

As the third millennium begins to unfold, it is truly heartening to see increasing numbers of pastors and parish priests offering regular opportunities for the churched and the unchurched to experience the Healing Christ. Church leaders, lay and clergy, now have access to excellent resources for being more faithful in this previously neglected area of Christian ministry.

The central focus of this book underscores a well-balanced personal lifestyle, with strong emphasis on the spiritual component. This book is not to be a Band-Aid for temporary relief of whatever comes along that makes us uncomfortable; rather, as Jesus demonstrated in his life and ministry, personal healing is a gift from God and a sign of God's grace inviting the healed ones to live every day in the kingdom of God. As Jesus said to his disciples: "Cure the sick who are there, and say to them, 'The kingdom of God has come near to you'" (Luke 10:9, NRSV).

Because Jesus loved the whole person, his goal was to help each one he met to be whole and healthy in body, mind, and spirit and in relationships. To experience relief from a specific physical illness and then not live a more faithful life in one's personal relationship with God and others indicates unhealthiness still exists. To be forgiven of personal sin and yet continue in a lifestyle that abuses the body, the mind, and other people is a sure sign of continuing sickness. To work at the discipline of maintaining physical fitness and mental alertness without regard to one's spirituality is to be less than whole and healthy. In his excellent book *Anchoring Your Well Being,* Dr. Howard Clinebell reminds us that

> Jesus highlights the purpose of his ministry: "I came that they may have life, and have it abundantly" (John 10:10). The New English Bible translates this Greek phrase as "life . . . in all its fullness." The abundant life or life in all its fullness is what is called spiritually empowered "well-being," "wholeness," or "wellness" in the contemporary language. . . . The fundamental purpose of the Christian life is to enable people to develop lifestyles of spiritually empowered wholeness throughout their life journeys and to help create a society in which life in all its fullness is possible for all members of the human family.[2]

I heartily affirm and support the healing professions and the medical sciences. Without doubt God uses medicine, hospitals, and various psychological therapies for our good health; however, our total health needs require receptivity to the best spiritual care and to living a healthy lifestyle. As a wise family doctor once said, "God is our primary physician, and all the doctors on earth are junior partners."

One of the most exciting developments in the healing arts is the demonstrated proof that religious faith significantly affects the healing process. Current medical investigation indicates that faith in God, who cares deeply and personally about each of us helps us, heal faster with less pain and less medication. Practicing physician Dale A. Matthews is a credible exponent of the faith factor. He is convinced,

> based on the research data we now have on hand, that your doctor could—from a strictly scientific point of view—recommend religious involvement [in a faith community] to improve your chances of being able to
> - stay healthy and avoid life-threatening and disabling diseases like cancer and heart disease;
> - recover faster and with fewer complications if you do develop a serious illness;
> - live longer;
> - encounter life-threatening and terminal illnesses with greater peacefulness and less pain;
> - avoid mental illnesses like depression and anxiety and cope more effectively with stress;
> - steer clear of problems with alcohol, drugs, tobacco;
> - enjoy a happier marriage and family life;
> - find a greater sense of meaning and purpose in life.[3]

We must acknowledge that maintaining good health throughout a lifetime or recovering completely from illnesses are mysteries beyond human understanding. For those who try to answer the unanswerable questions, Albert E. Day, a pastor of a generation ago, offers a word of caution based on his research in healing ministry:

There are not a few persons who find it difficult to live with mystery and to accept the arrival of new questions; but as one has said, "The postulate of all scholarly investigation is the nagging experience of mystery. . . . Our answers will not banish all mystery, but they will honor the God involved in the mystery and will help men and women to an ever-growing comprehension and experience of God's love and power.

Of this much we are certain: some for whom we pray will experience a physical healing which could not otherwise have been their happy lot; others will enter into a blessed, conscious comradeship with God; and all will know that the church and its ministers deeply care for them, feel their pains, share their griefs. The church will become "a fellowship of those who bear the mark of pain," which is, strangely enough, a fellowship of unique joy.[4]

In this book I invite you to focus on thirty meditations based on the healing stories of Jesus in the four Gospels. I intentionally quote the entire healing story in each meditation from the Contemporary English Version (CEV), published by the American Bible Society in 1995. I find the CEV to be fresh, easy to read, and quite understandable. The CEV has been described as a "'user-friendly' translation . . . that can be *read aloud* without stumbling, *heard* without misunderstanding, and *listened to* with enjoyment and appreciation, because the language is contemporary."[5]

Throughout this book I do quote briefly from other translations for comparison and clarity. I encourage readers to compare the CEV scripture texts to other versions. Unless they can read the New Testament in the original Greek and Aramaic languages, English-speaking people thankfully rely upon a host of English translations to allow the Word of God to penetrate, communicate, heal, inspire, guide, and take residence in our hearts and lives.

I have tried to distinguish between the name "Jesus" and the title "Christ." The name "Jesus," from a Hebrew word for "the Lord saves" or "Jehovah is salvation," was given to Joseph by an angel in a dream before Jesus's birth (see Matt. 1:18-25). In the four Gospels, Jesus is fully human, experiencing and expressing a variety of human emotions, feelings, and relationships with other people. Because his relationship with God was so intimate and special, Jesus called God his heavenly Father or Abba (Daddy). The primary mission of Jesus in his adult life was to do the will of God and to proclaim the coming of God's kingdom by preaching, teaching, and healing. Consequently, God was quite able to work in and through the flesh-and-blood Jesus to give people hope, help, healing, wholeness, well-being, and salvation.

I use the title "Christ" (from the Greek word for "messiah" or "God's Anointed One)" in referring to Jesus after he came back from the grave on Easter. From that point on he was no longer confined to his physical body or to being in only one place at a time. His followers began to understand that Jesus truly was the long-awaited Messiah. Interchangeably I use the terms *Holy Spirit, Spirit of Christ, Healing Christ, Spirit of the Living God, Spirit of Jesus,* and *Risen Christ* when referring to God's empowering, loving, healing, saving presence yesterday, today, and in all of God's tomorrows.

If you are ready to give your heart's and mind's attention to the spiritual dimension of your life and to adjust your lifestyle for maximum health, then I invite you to use this book as a personal devotional guide along with the suggested Bible readings. You could also invite a small group of friends to use this book individually and then get together for mutual sharing, accountability, and prayer.

From my personal experiences, I know that you can trust the Holy Spirit and trust the process whereby you grow in relationship with God and become conformed to the mind and Spirit of Christ. Practicing the spiritual discipline of having time alone with God every day

  bonds your connection with God;

  reminds you that you are not alone, that the Risen Christ is with you;

  helps you manage stress better;

19

- ❦ centers and strengthens the foundations of your faith;

- ❦ gives your mind, body, and spirit "time out" for relaxation and re-creation;

- ❦ orders your priorities;

- ❦ invites the Holy Spirit to move, act, and intervene in your life as you pray about everything and anything;

- ❦ gives the Healing Christ the opportunity to touch and to heal you at all levels of your being and in every area of your life;

- ❦ inspires and motivates you to pray more intentionally for your family, friends, and strangers;

- ❦ makes you more aware of the peace of Christ that surpasses all human understanding.

As the apostle Paul wrote, "Let the same mind be in you that was in Christ Jesus" (Phil. 2:5, NRSV).

James K. Wagner
Galloway, Ohio

SOME WAYS TO USE THIS BOOK

For Private Devotions

Wisdom gleaned from faithful Christians throughout the history of the church clearly and without exception encourages all followers of Jesus to be purposeful, intentional, and disciplined in setting aside time to be alone with God. When we do this, even sporadically, we know firsthand the blessings and benefits that accompany times of private devotion. So why not every day in a regular way? Consider this insightful observation by Albert E. Day, founder of the Disciplined Order of Christ.

> The spiritual power of the church depends not upon complicated organization or creative administration, important as these are; not upon eloquent preaching nor adequate theology, valuable as they are; not even upon unlimited financial resources.
>
> What the church primarily needs today, as always, is the presence of God-conscious, God-centered Christians. Even a few here and there would greatly help a church confronted by the chaos of this age.[6]

This book's design gives a workable format, a simple structure, to your private moments with God. Keep in mind this is not the same as, nor does it take the place of, your time spent in church for worship services and other corporate gatherings for praise and prayer. You have several options in using this book as a personal devotional guide. Each one is based on the *lectio divina* tradition in Christian spiritual formation (see pages 25–26). You may want to separate the bookmark from the cover of the book, then use it to locate your page and to keep in front of you these helpful guidelines for time alone with God.

Option One. Follow the book's sequence for the thirty healing scripture themes. Each New Testament healing story is printed in full, followed by a focused commentary by the author plus a related quotation from another source called "A Reading to Think About." The "Personal Reflection" section encourages you to write down your thoughts, feelings, and responses.

Option Two. Follow the six steps outlined in "Getting Up Close and Personal with the Healing Stories of Jesus" (see pages 27–28). This pattern gives you more freedom in scripture selection and in your personal devotional style.

Option Three. Keep a personal journal or notebook. Some readers may find the writing space too limited in the "Personal Reflection" sections.

Option Four. Move at your own pace, perhaps taking six or seven days for each of the thirty meditations. To use this book on a daily basis, focus on only one of the "Personal Reflection" guidelines each day. A small dose every day is a more effective Christian formational way.

If setting aside time every day for meditation and prayer is an unfamiliar spiritual discipline, begin at a comfortable level. Start with a minimum of fifteen minutes each day for one week. Then review the experience. Do you need to relocate your private space? Is your time of day or night suitable? What did not work for you? What worked well and turned out to be positive for you? Would it help to discuss this devotional practice with a trusted friend?

If you are still harboring the notion that perhaps you are too busy to follow one of these plans, look at the hectic, stressful, fast-paced life of Jesus. He felt compelled, even driven, to spend time alone with God each day. His contemporary disciples could well follow his excellent example: "After [Jesus] had dismissed the crowds, he went up the mountain by himself to pray. When evening came, he was there alone" (Matt. 14:23, NRSV). Jesus wants us to experience for ourselves not only the inner peace that is beyond human understanding but also a liberated life, a God-centered life, a God-directed life, a life whose security does not depend on things that can be taken away.

For Small Group Study and Discussion

One person may lead or coordinate the entire study, or group members may take turns leading from session to session. Group leaders need to be flexible and sensitive to the personal situation of each group member, especially in times of sharing and praying.

To foster group participation, ownership, and accountability in this spiritual formation experience, invite the group members to covenant (agree)

> ❦ to be present for all sessions;

> ❦ to meet once a week, if at all possible;

> ❦ to pray for one another daily;

> ❦ to read, study, and meditate on the assigned material in preparation for each meeting;

> ❦ to express disagreements and various opinions in an atmosphere of mutual support;

> ❦ to come to each group meeting with a loving heart, an open mind, and a teachable spirit;

> ❦ to saturate each session with prayer, allowing the focus of prayers to arise from the felt needs and life situations of the moment;

> ❦ to set time limits for each meeting (no less than one hour or more than two).

Let the group decide which study pattern to use. You may choose between the following options:

a. follow the thirty healing scripture themes and the printed format; or

b. select healing stories randomly from the Scripture Index and then follow the six steps listed in "Getting Up Close and Personal with the Healing Stories of Jesus."

At each group session, consider these questions:

1. What insights or questions came to you during your study of this scripture passage?
2. What were some of your thoughts and feelings during your reflection and meditation times?
3. What challenges and changes did this healing story prompt you to make in your life?

Your shared times together are opportunities to discover the mind and Spirit of Christ in your midst. If your group would like to continue meeting after completing this book, you are invited to review the Resources for other study materials.

PRAYING THE SCRIPTURES: LECTIO DIVINA

Lectio divina is a way of praying the Holy Scriptures and listening to God. A divine and human dialogue is desired. God speaks to us. We listen and respond. We speak to God, who listens and responds. In this devotional guide we will follow the *lectio divina* approach to the suggested biblical passages.

> Our inner posture is one of a listening heart filled with an unhurried expectation that God has a message to convey especially suited to our condition and circumstance. We read and ruminate with the ears of our heart open, alert to connections the Spirit may reveal between the passage and our life situation. We ask, "What are you saying to me today, Lord? What am I to hear in this story, parable, prophecy?" Listening in this way requires an attitude of patient receptivity in which we let go of our own agendas and open ourselves to God's shaping purpose.[7]

Here is how *lectio divina* works. We enter God's Word through four movements:[8]

> The first movement is *lectio,* or reading. We prepare ourselves for God by taking time to quiet our bodies and minds. We open our Bible expecting God's word to address us, and we read with openness of heart and readiness to respond.

In the thirty meditations in this book, "Centering Prayer" and "Holy Scripture" reading correspond with the first movement, or *lectio.*

> The second movement is *meditatio,* or reflecting. We engage the text with our minds. . . . We search for relevant meanings, applications, and insights. We involve ourselves imaginatively in the text. . . . We seek to hear what God wants to communicate to us today.

The sections titled "Focus on the Scripture" and "A Reading to Think About" relate to the second movement, or *meditatio.*

> The third movement is *oratio,* or response. We move from thinking about God to conversing with God. Reflection on the scripture gives way to and guides the exchanges of a living relationship. Thought turns to prayer as we address God personally. Dialogue ensues as we respond in all honesty to what we feel God is saying to us and listen to God's response. . . . We pour out our love for God in adoration and intercession and experience the gift of a renewed spirit.

The "Personal Reflection" sections in the thirty meditations become the third movement, or *oratio.*

> The fourth movement is *contemplatio,* or rest. . . . We move from conversation with God to communion with God. We relax our efforts to actively meditate and pray. We let God be God in us. Our sole desire is to be one with our Lord, to live our lives today as [God's] love is leading us.

The section listed as "Resting in God's Presence" in each meditation is *contemplatio* and can be the most illuminating and renewing of the four movements in *lectio divina.*

The ongoing process of spiritual formation and transformation in and by God's Word enlightens our understanding of Paul's personal testimony: "It is no longer I who live, but it is Christ who lives in me" (Gal. 2:20, NRSV). Each time we open our Bible in the intimacy of God's presence, we are thankful and sensitive to the basic rhythm of *lectio divina:* reading, reflecting, responding, resting.

GETTING UP CLOSE AND PERSONAL WITH THE HEALING STORIES OF JESUS

Note to Reader: This devotional plan provides an alternative to reading the thirty printed themes and healing stories sequentially. This devotional plan gives you the option of selecting various healing passages from the Scripture Index. Allow at least thirty minutes (more would be better) to pray through these six steps.

Step 1: Getting Started

- ❧ Gather your Bible and a notebook for writing personal responses and journaling.

- ❧ Locate a quiet place. Take several long, slow breaths in a relaxed posture that is comfortable for you.

- ❧ Offer a prayer of thanks for this unrepeatable moment in your life, and ask God to disconnect you from any thoughts that might prevent you from giving God 100 percent of your attention.

Step 2: Unpacking God's Word (Lectio)

- ❧ Select a healing story in the Bible.

- ❧ Read the scripture slowly at least twice, silently or aloud.

- ❧ Write out the specific illness or problem in this story.

🌿 List various factors that contributed to the healing.

🌿 Where in this story do you find faith?

🌿 Write down any questions you may have about this story.

Step 3: Reflecting on God's Word (Meditatio)

🌿 Can you identify with this story in any way?

🌿 How is God speaking to you through this story?

🌿 What are some possible challenges and changes being suggested for your personal situation?

🌿 Be specific. Write down whatever comes to you.

Step 4: Listening to God (Oratio)

🌿 Continue quietly to center your thoughts on God in a trusting, receptive, expectant manner.

🌿 Be still and listen . . . listen . . . listen.

🌿 Reread the selected passage.

🌿 Record whatever comes to you.

🌿 Do not hurry God or cut short your listening.

Step 5: Resting in God (Contemplatio)

🌿 Relax your efforts to pray and meditate actively. Put aside your personal agenda.

🌿 Simply enjoy being in God's presence. Allow God's love to hold you and enfold you.

Step 6: Naming Your Next Step

🌿 When you are ready to move on, offer a prayer of thanks for these precious, special moments.

🌿 Ask for God's grace, guidance, and encouragement to help you act upon any direction that may have come to you during your time alone with God. Name possible next steps.

🌿 Depend on God's faithfulness to you.

🌿 Go now in peace for the peace of Christ goes with you!

1

JESUS THE HEALER

Centering Prayer

Thanks be to thee, O Lord Jesus Christ, for all the benefits which thou hast given us; for all the pains and insults which thou hast borne for us. O most merciful Redeemer, friend, and brother, may we know thee more clearly, love thee more dearly, and follow thee more nearly, for thine own sake. Amen.[9]

Holy Scripture

MATTHEW 4:23-25

Jesus went all over Galilee, teaching in the Jewish meeting places and preaching the good news about God's kingdom. He also healed every kind of disease and sickness. News about him spread all over Syria, and people with every kind of sickness or disease were brought to him. Some of them had a lot of demons in them, others were thought to be crazy, and still others could not walk. But Jesus healed them all.

Large crowds followed Jesus from Galilee and the region around the ten cities known as Decapolis. They also came from Jerusalem, Judea, and from across the Jordan River.

 Focus on the Scripture

When defining health and healing, we take our cue from the demonstrated ministries of Jesus Christ. In the New Testament health connotes more than the absence of disease. Although Jesus was primarily interested in each person's having a healthy relationship with God, he loved the whole person and facilitated health and wholeness in spirit, body, mind, and human relationships. Add to the four areas of healing the ultimate healing of the Christian in the resurrection of Christ after the body's death.

In *Letters on the Healing Ministry*, Albert E. Day, a pioneer in holistic healing ministry in the former Methodist Church, wrote that health is a "combination of harmonious relationships, spiritual vitality, psychological maturity, and physical wellness."[10]

The purpose of Christ's healing ministry is to help people restore and maintain a healthy balance among the body, the mind, the spirit, and personal relationships. The healing of nations and the healing of planet Earth (environmental concerns) are also significant issues in health and wholeness ministry.

Frequently people ask questions about God's will in the ongoing struggle between health and sickness. Does our Creator God truly desire good health for all humanity? The following evidence affirms the answer of an undoubted yes:

 ❧ God's good creation as described in the Genesis 1–2;

 ❧ the body's natural ability to heal itself;

 ❧ Jesus' intentional, compassionate healing ministry;

 ❧ the continuing research and newly discovered resources of the health-care professions.

Clearly God has unlimited ways to enhance human health. However, for the Christian the primary resource is the abiding, loving, living presence of the Healing Christ. These spiritual therapies help us stay connected with Christ, the source of life and health: prayer, faith, music, anointing with oil, laying on hands, liturgy, Bible study, the sacraments, special places, and the love of caring persons. The Holy Spirit can use all of the above as signs pointing us to Christ and as helpful ways to get us in touch with Christ our Savior, our Lord, and our Healer.

Affirm in your heart and offer a prayer of thanksgiving for the presence of the Healing Christ in your life this very moment. As you make room in your daily life for time alone with God, you will know the truth and the reality of this passage where the Risen Christ says to the faithful, "Listen! I am standing at the door, knocking; if you hear my voice and open the door, I will come in to you and eat with you, and you with me" (Rev. 3:20, NRSV).

A Reading to Think About

BY ALBERT E. DAY

Whenever we talk about spiritual healing, we are . . . not suggesting that some miracle is necessary to bring God on the scene, or that some natural laws are violated by the insurgence of divine pity into a situation from which God has until that moment been absent. We are only, but imperfectly, saying that the God always present, but limited by humanity's ignorance or unbelief or self-will, has been given a free hand in humanity's life. We are saying that God has been invited to reign in a life where self has been on the throne; that God's kingdom has become more truly a reality in that life; that that person has entered the kingdom of God.[11]

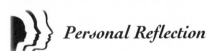 *Personal Reflection*

What is God saying to you in this story?

1. Carefully read and reread the scripture passage. Write down any thoughts, ideas, and questions that may come to you. Do not hurry.

2. Focus on one verse, Matthew 4:24: "People with every kind of sickness or disease were brought to him. . . . But Jesus healed them all." What an awesome statement! That statement means he can also heal you of every kind of unhealthiness. Invite the risen, compassionate Spirit of Jesus to love you as you love him and to touch the unhealed areas of your life.

3. Thankful people are healthier people. Take your time as you enter into this litany of thanksgiving with prayer:

❧ Thank God for creating planet Earth with everything needed for the welfare and well-being of humankind.

❧ Thank God for creating your body with built-in systems of renewal and regeneration.

❧ Thank God for your doctor, your dentist, your optometrist, your nurse, your counselor, your therapist, and others (by name) in the health-care professions whom you call on for help and healing.

❧ Thank God for the Healing Christ who actively participates in your quest for health and wholeness in body, mind, spirit, and in all your relationships.

❧ Thank God for the healing love you have experienced in times of past personal illness and be open to God's therapies in dealing with any present or future unhealthiness.

4. For what else do you give thanks to God, the giver of every good and perfect gift?

5. As you launch out on this spiritual-formation experience, what questions and personal issues do you bring with you?

Caring Prayer for Others

Pray for someone you know who does not know Christ and who needs the kind of health that only comes from the all-sufficient Christ.

Resting in God's Presence

Now put aside your personal agenda and simply relax, basking in the warmth and healing light of God's love.

Go forth from this special place knowing that the grace and peace of Christ go with you!

2

DO YOU WANT TO BE HEALED?

Centering Prayer

Disconnect me, O Christ, from all that prevents my connection with you. Right now, I want to give you my complete attention. Amen.

Holy Scripture

JOHN 5:1-9,14-15

Later, Jesus went to Jerusalem for another Jewish festival. In the city near the sheep gate was a pool with five porches, and its name in Hebrew was Bethzatha.

Many sick, blind, lame, and crippled people were lying close to the pool. [*Author's note:* They were waiting for the water to be stirred, because an angel from the Lord would sometimes come down and stir it. The first person to get into the pool after that would be healed.]

Beside the pool was a man who had been sick for thirty-eight years. When Jesus saw the man and realized that he had been crippled for a long time, he asked him, "Do you want to be healed?" The man answered, "Lord, I don't have anyone to put me in the pool when the water is stirred up. I try to get in, but someone else always gets there first."

Jesus told him, "Pick up your mat and walk!" Right then the man was healed. He picked up his mat and started walking around. The day on which this happened was a Sabbath. . . .

Later, Jesus met the man in the temple and told him, "You are now well. But don't sin anymore or something worse might happen to you." The man left and told the leaders that Jesus was the one who had healed him.

 ## Focus on the Scripture

A rather odd question Jesus asked this man, or is it? "Tell me, do you want to be healed?" Actually this is not a strange or inappropriate concern on Jesus' part.

Some people say they want to get better but don't do much about it. Sickness becomes their lifestyle. Sometimes people with this attitude are accused of "enjoying poor health." One doctor asks his long-suffering, chronically ill patients a tough question: What personal benefits would you have to give up if you became well again?

Some people may want to get well but have convinced themselves that they are incurable. So why seek medical or spiritual help? The disabled man in the story believed there was only one cure, the healing water, or hydrotherapy, of the Pool of Bethzatha. That avenue was not open to him, however, because he had no friends to help him get there ahead of the crowd. Is this not a picture of a severely discouraged human being who has given up all hope of ever getting well again? Could this explain why Jesus' first words dealt with the man's hopelessness?

When Jesus entered this man's situation, he first offered hope. Without hope, spiritual or mental or physical therapy will not be very effective. The man in the story would have been satisfied with just being able to walk again, but God's healing agenda is always much more comprehensive than restored physical well-being.

This man received healing three different ways: His mental outlook became positive; his physical problems evaporated as he began to walk again; and he experienced a new relationship with God as his sins were forgiven. My hunch is that Jesus also helped him deal with his resentment and bitterness toward those who would never lend a hand when needed. Withholding forgiveness can block the healing process.

The question Jesus asked also is critical for you if you should ever become totally discouraged, nursing a negative attitude around the clock. Attitude, as James Moore has wisely commented, is the mind's paintbrush. It can color any situation.[12] Call on the presence of the Healing Christ, especially during those times when you begin to lose hope and need an attitude adjustment along with restored health.

A Reading to Think About

BY FLORA SLOSSON WUELLNER

When we have allowed God's healing light to enter us fully, there is a change within us. Some of these changes come slowly, others swiftly. Some may come almost simultaneously, whereas others may come at long intervals. We cannot tell in which order the changes will come. Sometimes we will be immediately conscious of inner changes, and at other times we may be aware of nothing happening on the surface, but great transformation is occurring at levels far below the conscious awareness.[13]

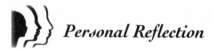 *Personal Reflection*

What is God saying to you in this story?

1. Carefully read and reread the scripture passage. Write down any thoughts, ideas, and questions that may come to you. Do not hurry.

2. Name the specific illness or problem in this story and list all factors that seemed to work together for healing.

3. It might be helpful for you to name some of the personal benefits you receive when you get sick. Keep in mind that you lose these when your health returns.

4. Recall a time in your life when you became very discouraged. How did that feel? How did that discouragement impact your daily life? What factors helped you move through your discouragement?

5. If you are discouraged right now—feeling no hope, having no positive answers—take courage from this healing story. Invite the Healing Christ into your hopeless situation. In conversational prayer, with nothing held back, lay out your situation and feelings completely to Christ, your Savior and Healer. You may need to deal with the key question: Do you

want to be healed? Record any personal thoughts, feelings, and promptings of the Holy Spirit.

Caring Prayer for Others

Name someone you know who has given up hope and who may be refusing help. Pray for that child of God as God's Spirit leads you.

Resting in God's Presence

Now put aside your personal agenda and simply relax, basking in the warmth and healing light of God's love.

Go forth from this special place knowing that the grace and peace of Christ go with you!

 **3**

DON'T GIVE UP!

Centering Prayer

O God, my Creator and Re-Creator, may the transforming power of your gracious gospel be at work in my life this day and every day, as I come to you in the name that is above all other names, in the name of Jesus. Amen.

Holy Scripture

MARK 7:24-30

Jesus left and went to the region near the city of Tyre, where he stayed in someone's home. He did not want people to know he was there, but they found out anyway. A woman whose daughter had an evil spirit in her heard where Jesus was. And right away she came and knelt down at his feet. The woman was Greek and had been born in the part of Syria known as Phoenicia. She begged Jesus to force the demon out of her daughter. But Jesus said, "The children must first be fed! It isn't right to take away their food and feed it to dogs."

The woman replied, "Lord, even dogs eat the crumbs that children drop from the table."

Jesus answered, "That's true! You may go now. The demon has left your daughter." When the woman got back home, she found her child lying on the bed. The demon had gone. (See also Matt. 15:21-28.)

Focus on the Scripture

This unusual healing story has been described as one of the most difficult as well as one of the most moving, thoughtful incidents in the life of Jesus. Because a surface reading of this text makes little sense, the tendency is not to take it seriously or to skip over it.

Several curious details set the stage for this intriguing conversation between Jesus and the Phoenician woman. First of all Jesus is not on Jewish turf. Secondly he does not want anyone to know where he is. Why? Could it be that he simply needed some personal time for rest and recuperation from the unrelenting pressures of his ministry? "Yet he could not escape notice" (Mark 7:24, NRSV). Somehow word got out that Jesus was there, and immediately a Greek woman found him and begged him to help her daughter back home who had an evil spirit in her. This was not the only time a Gentile asked Jesus for personal assistance. However, it is the only recorded story informing us that Jesus initially resisted the request. How should we interpret this strange remark about feeding children and not feeding dogs? It seems a bit unkind, yet notice that Jesus did not shut the door on this woman; rather, he was reminding her that his primary mission was to the children of Israel. In Matthew's version of this story, Jesus explained to the woman, "I was sent only to the people of Israel! They are like a flock of lost sheep" (Matt. 15:24).

Jews of that period sometimes referred to Gentiles as "dogs." This distraught mother, however, would not be put off and responded with words that impressed Jesus. She said, "Lord, even dogs eat the crumbs that children drop from the table." Jesus answered, "That's true! You may go now. The demon has left your daughter" (Mark 7:28-29).

What appears to be a clever argument that resolved in the woman's favor turns out to be a prophetic word, because the gospel, originally intended for the Jews, was rejected by Judaism and took hold and flourished in the hearts, minds, and lives of Gentiles after the Day of Pentecost (see Acts 2).

Was Jesus simply testing this woman's faith? Possibly. Was Jesus using this teaching moment to plant the seeds for the gospel's future harvest? Possibly.

Other questions arise from this story. Jesus cured the child. The demon left her, but we do not learn what manner of healing Jesus used to expel the evil spirit.[14] Although this story raises several unanswered questions, we can praise God for Jesus' power and authority over evil and thank Mark and Matthew for including this special healing moment in their Gospel records.

A Reading to Think About

BY ALBERT E. DAY

The power of the kingdom, in the life of one in whom God reigns and has a free hand, may operate directly upon another who is ill even though that other person is not yet wholly committed to God. That seems to be what happened to Jesus. He was a kingdom man. His will was "to do the will of God in heaven." If ever God reigned without a rival in a human being, it was in the life of Jesus of Nazareth. So the power of the kingdom, which is the power of God, operated in him and through him upon the lives of others.[15]

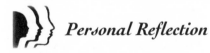 *Personal Reflection*

What is God saying to you in this story?

1. Carefully read and reread the scripture passage. Write down any thoughts, ideas, and questions that may come to you. Do not hurry.

2. Name the specific illness or problem in this story and list all factors that seemed to work together for healing.

3. Those of us who actively participate in churches tend to forget that God loves the whole world; that God's grace, mercy, and salvation include everyone and exclude no one (John 3:16). Reflect on your own interaction or lack of interaction with non-Christians. Remind yourself that the only gospel they may know is the gospel they see in you and in your lifestyle. How would you describe the gospel according to you and your living habits?

4. The nameless woman in this story refused to give up even though it seemed impossible to find healing for her child. Name some of your personal worries, anxieties, concerns, or problems that seem impossible to resolve and work out.

5. Take your impossible situation to God in prayer: O God of unlimited possibilities, even as the Phoenician woman came to Jesus with faith and trust that Jesus could heal her daughter back home, so I come to you right now, praying in the name of Jesus, asking for your help with these seemingly impossible situations that I face today. [*Name those you listed in number 4 above.*] Thank you, caring God. Amen.

Now quiet yourself and listen. Allow your spiritual ears to hear what God may be saying and suggesting to you. When you are ready to move on, thank God for this special time together and for the courage and guidance to act on some possible solutions.

Caring Prayer for Others

Think of someone you know who is living with an impossible situation, someone who is discouraged and about to give up. Pray tenderly, lovingly, thankfully for that child of God.

Resting in God's Presence

Now put aside your personal agenda and simply relax, basking in the warmth and healing light of God's love.

Go forth from this special place knowing that the grace and peace of Christ go with you.

 *4*

BENT OUT OF SHAPE

Centering Prayer

Just as your word, gracious and caring God, conveyed power, compassion, and healing in biblical times, so may your word in this hour speak to my weaknesses, protect me from evil, and straighten out the bent places of my heart, mind, body, and spirit. Amen.

Holy Scripture

LUKE 13:10-17

One Sabbath, Jesus was teaching in a Jewish meeting place, and a woman was there who had been crippled by an evil spirit for eighteen years. She was completely bent over and could not straighten up. When Jesus saw the woman, he called her over and said, "You are now well." He placed his hands on her, and right away she stood up straight and praised God.

The man in charge of the meeting place was angry because Jesus had healed someone on the Sabbath. So he said to the people, "Each week has six days when we can work. Come and be healed on one of those days, but not on the Sabbath."

The Lord replied, "Are you trying to fool someone? Won't any one of you untie your ox or donkey and lead it out to drink on a Sabbath? This woman belongs to the family of Abraham, but Satan has kept her bound for eighteen years. Isn't it right to set her free on the Sabbath?" Jesus' words made his enemies ashamed.

But everyone else in the crowd was happy about the wonderful things he was doing.

 Focus on the Scripture

At first reading, this story has the familiar ring of the time when Jesus was teaching in a synagogue on the Sabbath and he was verbally assaulted by a man with an evil spirit, which disrupted the meeting. (See meditation 13, "Evil Confronted," based on Luke 4:31-37 and Mark 1:21-28.) There are, however, differing details in this heartwarming healing incident.

A nameless woman with severe curvature of the spine was present that day in the back of the room. Was she trying to get Jesus' attention? No. Did she attempt to disrupt the meeting? No. She was just there, doing what faithful Jews do on the Sabbath, attending the synagogue service. Having been crippled for eighteen years, she probably had given up hope of ever standing straight again.

The scene changes quickly in verse 12. When Jesus saw the woman, his compassionate, sensitive heart would not let him continue with his intended teaching. So Jesus interrupted the meeting with an invitation to the obviously surprised woman. He called her over to him.

Reading between the lines, you can hear her questioning why Jesus would pay any attention to her. But she did have a choice in the matter: She could slip away quietly and avoid the embarrassing attention or she could come forward, hoping against hope that maybe, just maybe, the famous rabbi could help her. Then she heard him say directly to her those incredible words: "You are now well."

Picture that moment in your mind: This called-out woman inching her way forward, trying to ignore the murmurings of the other people. Then, as a reinforcement of his healing word and as an affirmation to the astonished woman, Jesus physically touches her and instantly she becomes unbent and stands up, praising God.

Is this another healing story with a happy ending? For the cured woman, yes. For Jesus, no. Those who believe that people who help others are always appreciated and equally rewarded are soon disillusioned. Doing good is risky business. Jesus knew this, but it never stopped him. He did what he thought was right at the moment and accepted the consequences of his actions.

Traditional Jewish attitudes toward Sabbath rules and observances baffle most contemporary Christians. Yet we must remember that Jesus quite often was denounced and ridiculed for his behavior on the Sabbath. Repeatedly people accused him of disregarding the laws of Moses. This charge was among those that led to his crucifixion and death.

The reference to Satan in the story indicates the popular belief of the day that disabling conditions were linked to evil. People would inquire if physical infirmity and all kinds of sicknesses were signs of punishment or discipline from God. This story of the bent-over woman offers scriptural proof that the answer to that frequently raised question is no. The healing ministry of Jesus demonstrated again and again that all illness is to be confronted and overcome, regardless of the reasons causing the unhealthiness. God's will supports every effort to have healthy bodies, minds, spirits, and relationships.

A Reading to Think About

BY FRANCIS J. MOLONEY

It is remarkable just how much material in the Gospels gives us a rather startling vision of how Jesus related to women, and enables us to come closer to his attitude to woman as such. . . .

There was an extraordinarily deep inner peace and freedom in Jesus of Nazareth, which shows that he was ultimately free from all culturally, historically and even religiously conditioned constraints and prejudices. This has been made particularly clear through Jesus' allowing himself to both touch and be touched by women of all conditions.[16]

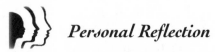 *Personal Reflection*

What is God saying to you in this story?

1. Carefully read and reread the scripture passage. Write down any thoughts, ideas, and questions that may come to you. Do not hurry.

2. Name the specific illness or problem in this story and list all factors that seemed to work together for healing.

3. Jesus got in trouble for doing something good in this story. Have you ever been put down, criticized, or not thanked for going out of your way to help someone? How did that feel? Rethink your interior motives for doing good works. Are you prepared to accept the consequences of your actions, even as Jesus did?

4. Recall how the elated woman contributed to the healing process. She heard Jesus directly invite her; she responded by going forward to him; she listened to his healing words

and felt his affirming touch as she stood up straight; then she praised God. Recall some personal healings in your own life. List some of the things you did to cooperate with God in the healing process. Praise and thank God!

5. Sometimes we get bent out of shape—in our relationships with others, by unkind and thoughtless words; in our personal attitudes toward life and living; in our immature, childish understandings of God. Jesus can and does want to help us. Close your eyes and visualize Jesus calling you forward and speaking to you those incredible words you have longed to hear, words that set you straight once more. Allow Jesus to touch the bent and broken places in your life and make you whole and healthy.

Caring Prayer for Others

Bring to Jesus in prayer anyone you know who may be bent out of shape and unable to enjoy full health—physically, mentally, spiritually, or in relationship with others.

Resting in God's Presence

Now put aside your personal agenda and simply relax, basking in the warmth and healing light of God's love.

Go forth from this special place knowing that the grace and peace of Christ go with you!

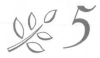 **5**

COMPASSION VERSUS POLICY

Centering Prayer

Free me, O God, from keeping back anything from you, thinking that you are too big or too busy to be concerned about everything, small and great, that happens in my life. Just as I am, I come to you now with my mask removed and my soul exposed to your merciful, healing, understanding presence. Amen.

Holy Scripture

LUKE 14:1-6

One Sabbath, Jesus was having dinner in the home of an important Pharisee, and everyone was carefully watching Jesus. All of a sudden a man with swollen legs stood up in front of him. Jesus turned and asked the Pharisees and the teachers of the Law of Moses, "Is it right to heal on the Sabbath?" But they did not say a word.

Jesus took hold of the man. Then he healed him and sent him away. Afterwards, Jesus asked the people, "If your son or ox falls into a well, wouldn't you pull him out right away, even on the Sabbath?" There was nothing they could say.

 Focus on the Scripture

Several details of this brief healing story catch our attention: the type of illness Jesus cured, the location of the healing, the day of the week on which the events took place. Most translations of Luke 14:2 indicate that the unknown man had dropsy, or swollen legs.

Dropsy is a shortened form of the Latin *hydropisis,* meaning "related to water." This sickness is characterized by excessive accumulation of fluid, usually in the legs, brought on by kidney or heart failure. It can be life-threatening. Today it is treatable but usually not curable.

We know nothing about this man, where he came from or why he was present at the dinner meeting. Since the setting is on the Sabbath and in the home of a very important Jewish official, this man with dropsy could well have been "planted" to force Jesus into yet another legal trap. Would Jesus ignore Sabbath rules prohibiting healing on the seventh day of the week, or would he put policy before compassion out of respect for his host?

Jesus knew what the Pharisee and his guests were thinking. Luke 14:1, NRSV, states, "They were watching him closely," meaning that they were scrutinizing Jesus carefully, analyzing his every move and word. Nevertheless Jesus chose to help the man who obviously was suffering and in much discomfort. Human need always took priority over community customs and regulations, according to Jesus. He decided to relieve the man of his suffering first, then debate with the teachers of the law of Moses. This consistent compassion characterized Jesus' entire public ministry.

The man cured of his dropsy by the physical touch and the healing faith of Jesus was sent away, no doubt glad to be well again and happy to be no longer a pawn in the Pharisees' game. Throughout this episode Jesus took the initiative in the ongoing debate on Sabbath rules. But according to Luke 14:4, 6, this was one of the few times his opponents were speechless. The dinner party got under way, and Jesus again took advantage of the moment to present more of his masterful teachings and insights (see Luke 14:7-24).

A Reading to Think About

BY ELTON TRUEBLOOD

The bold challenge of the Pharisees gave Christ a wonderful chance to deal with first principles, so far as vital religion is concerned. What He said was that it is not enough for God to be honored by using some particular linguistic or ceremonial formula. Anyone could do that, and he could, furthermore, do it with no change of heart whatever. He went on to point out that all ceremonies are [hu]man-made. . . .

Christ showed that tradition, being wholly [humanity's] doing, is never sufficient for true religion. It may not be based on intrinsic moral law at all. Indeed it is possible, by manipulating tradition, to subvert or to tone down a moral demand. Far from being apologetic or defensive, Christ immediately took the offensive and attacked the position of His adversaries. By this act He ruled out the possibility of compromise or appeasement. The issue was sharper than the Pharisees had expected it to be.[17]

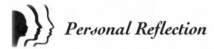 *Personal Reflection*

What is God saying to you in this story?

1. Carefully read and reread this scripture passage. Write down any thoughts, ideas, and questions that may come to you. Do not hurry.

2. Name the specific illness or problem in this story and list all factors that seemed to work together for healing.

3. The Gospel records of Jesus' ministry offer seven stories about his healing on the Sabbath day (three report the same incident). His guiding principle is stated in Mark 2:27: "People were not made for the good of the Sabbath. The Sabbath was made for the good of people." Rather than be overly critical of orthodox Judaism's multitude of Sabbath regulations, reflect on your own Sabbath observances. How do you keep the Lord's Day holy and different from the other six? Current medical research indicates that people who are active in their church, attending on a regular basis, receive health benefits and on the average live seven to fifteen years longer than those who do not have a faith community or church home. List some of the health benefits that you think could be derived from active church participation.

4. In this story Jesus' compassion went out to the man with the swollen legs. No human condition, illness, disease, or dysfunction is outside of Jesus' healing love and concern. If you are dealing with any type of unhealthiness in your life

today, name it here and give it to the Divine Physician for help and healing. Always remember it is okay to pray for yourself.

5. Compassion versus Policy: Examine those community customs and regulations (written as well as unwritten) that you allow to determine your thinking and your behavior. Are you aware of any time in your life when you have placed rigid policy above human compassion or social mores above God's morals? If so, consider what Jesus might say to you about that. Record your thoughts.

Caring Prayer for Others

Quiet yourself. Relax in God's presence. Thank God for this time together. Then ask God to bring into your mind names of persons for whom you can pray right now, especially those who seem to be long on living by rules and short on acting out of compassion.

Resting in God's Presence

Now put aside your personal agenda and simply relax, basking in the warmth and healing light of God's love.

Go forth from this special place knowing that the grace and peace of Christ go with you!

6

HEALING ANTICIPATED

Centering Prayer

O God, whose grace and mercy flow like an endless river from your great being, help me now to place myself in the path of your rushing love and limitless compassion, that I may find my spirit renewed. Amen.[18]

Holy Scripture

LUKE 5:12-16

Jesus came to a town where there was a man who had leprosy. When the man saw Jesus, he kneeled down to the ground in front of Jesus and begged, "Lord, you have the power to make me well, if only you wanted to."

Jesus put his hand on him and said, "I want to! Now you are well." At once the man's leprosy disappeared. Jesus told him, "Don't tell anyone about this, but go and show yourself to the priest. Offer a gift to the priest, just as Moses commanded, and everyone will know that you have been healed." News about Jesus kept spreading. Large crowds came to listen to him teach and to be healed of their diseases. But Jesus would often go to some place where he could be alone and pray. (See also Mark 1:40-45 and Matt. 8:1-4.)

Focus on the Scripture

The word *leprosy* appears frequently in the Bible and refers to a host of skin diseases, some mild and some quite severe. The unenlightened wisdom of that day heartlessly labeled all persons with unhealed, unhealthy skin as "lepers," calling them "unclean." Jesus had several encounters with persons who were diagnosed as having these dreaded disorders.

Because it was popularly believed that leprosy in all its various expressions was a contagious disease, lepers were social outcasts, not permitted to live in the villages, attend synagogue services, or participate in community activities. Lepers were labeled "the untouchables."

The leper in this story acted boldly. Knowing in his heart that Jesus had the power to heal him, he knelt down before the famous healer but did not know how Jesus might respond. Would Jesus chase him away as so many others had done or would Jesus want to help him?

Try to imagine how this man must have felt when Jesus not only touched him but also reassured him that he was now cured and no longer would anyone call him unclean.

To verify the healing, Jesus did what was expected. He sent the former leper to be examined by a priest, the only one who could authenticate healings and certify when people could return to a normal life in the Jewish community. To prove further that this healing was no hoax, Jesus instructed the man to honor the law of Moses and make a gift to the priest in the form of lambs, flour, and olive oil, the prescribed temple offering. Then everyone would know the truth. Jesus' insistence that the man see a temple priest immediately is a wise word to you when you or a loved one experiences personal healing by the grace, compassion, and power of God. Today, rather than going to a temple priest, you can make an appointment with your doctor to verify the healing. Then give God the glory.

A Reading to Think About

BY FRANK B. STANGER

As one seeks healing, there must be an eager expectancy, the attitude of an active faith. Never must a seeker think in terms of failure. Always there is the anticipation of God fulfilling what [God] has already promised. . . . I have learned in my healing ministries that this matter of anticipatory faith is crucial. I have not known of a case where this kind of faith was present, without any doubts whatever, when healing did not result. Far too often a person confesses that he or she thought there was genuine faith, but actually there were damaging inward doubts.[19]

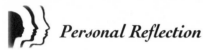 *Personal Reflection*

What is God saying to you in this story?

1. Carefully read and reread the scripture passage. Write down any thoughts, ideas, and questions that may come to you. Do not hurry.

2. Name the specific illness or problem in this story and list all factors that seemed to work together for healing.

3. Jesus treated all he met as persons of worth. No one was outside God's compassion, even those labeled as outcasts, sinners, and untouchables. Do you know people identified with such labels in your community, church, family? What is your attitude and behavior toward these human beings?

4. Frank B. Stanger states that anticipatory faith is crucial in healing. Recall healings in your life. Did you anticipate recovery? Did you pray with expectancy of something good to happen? Did God bless you in ways different from what you had expected? What does this anticipatory faith mean for your personal health and wholeness today and in the future?

5. Ponder Luke 5:15-16, being open to a message for you: "Large crowds came to listen to [Jesus] teach and to be healed of their diseases. But Jesus would often go to some place where he could be alone and pray." When you achieve some measure of success, when you are on the receiving end of complimentary words, when what you have to offer to others is effective and appreciated, what is your response? To whom do you give the credit? Do you, like Jesus, go to a place where you can be alone and pray?

Caring Prayer for Others

After naming some of the "untouchables" in your personal world, tenderly pray for each one, examine your attitude toward each one, and be open to Christ's word of direction for you.

Resting in God's Presence

Now put aside your personal agenda and simply relax, basking in the warmth and healing light of God's love.

Go forth from this special place knowing that the grace and peace of Christ go with you!

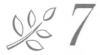 **7**

THE GRACE OF GRATITUDE

Centering Prayer

O God, from whom comes every good and perfect gift, grant me one thing more: the gift of a grateful heart, an appreciative and thankful attitude. Amen.

Holy Scripture

LUKE 17:11-19

On his way to Jerusalem, Jesus went along the border between Samaria and Galilee. As he was going into a village, ten men with leprosy came toward him. They stood at a distance and shouted, "Jesus, Master, have pity on us!"

Jesus looked at them and said, "Go show yourselves to the priests."

On their way they were healed. When one of them discovered that he was healed, he came back, shouting praises to God. He bowed down at the feet of Jesus and thanked him. The man was from the country of Samaria.

Jesus asked, "Weren't ten men healed? Where are the other nine? Why was this foreigner the only one who came back to thank God?" Then Jesus told the man, "You may get up and go. Your faith has made you well."

Focus on the Scripture

This passage is not the only Gospel record of Jesus' interaction with persons diagnosed with leprosy. (See meditation 6, "Healing Anticipated," based on Luke 5:12-16, the story of the lone leper who came to Jesus.) Even though the term *leprosy* covered a multitude of skin diseases in biblical times, the community mind-set forbade these unfortunate human beings to mix with the general population. This attitude explains the statement in Luke 17:12-13: "They stood at a distance and shouted." For additional data on the separatist attitude toward lepers, see Leviticus 13:45-46 and Numbers 5:2.

The lepers asked for pity (some translations say "mercy") from Jesus, who did what they asked and instructed them to go immediately to show themselves to the priests. Notice the story says that they were healed (made clean) on their way to see the priest. This means the ten men, trusting the word of Jesus, headed for the temple for a priestly verification of their healing before they were cured. This faith-action speaks well for them. Before the lepers arrived in Jerusalem, all ten discovered that they were no longer leprous. Their skin was healthy once more.

The story then takes an interesting twist in reporting that only one of the ten men turned around and came back to say thank you to Jesus, commenting additionally, "The man was from the country of Samaria" (Luke 17:16). We cannot assume that all ten were Samaritans. Even though Jews and Samaritans did not mix socially, that probably did not apply to lepers who may have banded together just for survival regardless of their ethnic origin. Clearly Jesus, who refers to this man as a foreigner, was taken by surprise at his genuine appreciation as the man bowed down, thanked Jesus, and praised God.

Observe the strong, undeniable importance that Jesus placed on personal gratitude: "Weren't ten men healed? Where are the other nine? Why was this foreigner the only one who came back to thank God?" (Luke 17:17-18). We cannot overestimate the power of appreciation and thankfulness in the healing process and especially in healing the whole person. Thankful persons are healthier than unthankful persons. Extensive research in the area of stress and distress confirms the therapeutic nature of gratitude. Negative emotions and attitudes such as resentment, revenge, anger, hate, and jealousy debilitate the body's disease-controlling immune system; whereas the positive emotions and attitudes such as gratitude, thanksgiving, praise, forgiveness, and joy enhance health.

Obviously the nine thankless men only wanted a physical cure. The thankful tenth man, by praising God and demonstrating his genuine heartfelt appreciation, received physical healing plus more. God's agenda for our personal health plan includes the body, the mind, the spirit, and our relationships with others. This is why Jesus said to the man, "You may get up and go. Your faith has made you well." The Greek word for "well" also can be translated: cured, healed, saved, preserved, or made whole. Jesus was very pleased with the man's positive attitude and authentic gratitude.

A Reading to Think About

BY ADRIAN VAN KAAM AND SUSAN MUTO

Appreciation is the single most important disposition to be cultivated in our life and world today. The power of appreciation helps us to look at the directions for living offered by everyday events, good, bad, and indifferent, in a new way. . . . We are born to be appreciated and to become appreciative. We only need to flow with the grace of gratitude. Once this happens you will delight in your new-found appreciation of self, world, others, and their mysterious source. Appreciation will grow into a warm presence to the gifts in cosmos and creation as expressions of a divine generosity. You will exude care for all that is good.[20]

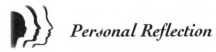 *Personal Reflection*

What is God saying to you in this story?

1. Carefully read and reread the scripture passage. Write down any thoughts, ideas, and questions that may come to you. Do not hurry.

2. Name the specific illness or problem in this story and list all factors that seemed to work together for healing.

3. The ten men stood at a distance, asking Jesus to help them, not knowing if they would be welcomed by him if they came any closer. Jesus did not insist that they come forward so that he could physically touch them. He respected their dignity and personal situations. Likewise today, the Healing Christ does not make uncomfortable demands. His sensitivity and caring meet us where we are and invite us to be receptive to God's total health care for each of us. Name your personal health needs. Then ask God to guide your next step toward wholeness in body, mind, spirit, and personal relationships.

4. Do you have difficulty saying thank you? Does your lifestyle reflect a grateful heart? What are some ways you could be

more open and sincere in expressing appreciation, especially to those who love you the most?

5. "Bless the Lord, O my soul, and do not forget all his benefits" (Ps. 103:2, NRSV). One way to do this is to make a mental list at the end of each day of at least ten good things that happened in your life. Recalling positive experiences will not only offset the things that did not go well but also will help you relax and get a restful night's sleep. What other things can you do to cultivate a lifelong attitude and practice of appreciation and thankfulness?

Caring Prayer for Others

Pray for persons you know who are not pleasant to be around because of their constant grumbling and complaining. Pray for the Holy Spirit to sweeten their spirit, adjust their attitude, and bless them in special ways.

Resting in God's Presence

Now put aside your personal agenda and simply relax, basking in the warmth and healing of God's love.

Go forth from this special place knowing that the grace and peace of Christ go with you!

8

FAITH-FULL FRIENDS

Centering Prayer

As a deer longs for flowing streams,
    so my soul longs for you, O God.
My soul thirsts for God,
    for the living God.
When shall I come and behold
    the face of God? . . .
By day the Lord commands his steadfast love,
    and at night his song is with me,
    a prayer to the God of my life (Ps. 42:1-2, 8, NRSV).

Holy Scripture

LUKE 5:17-26

One day some Pharisees and experts in the Law of Moses sat listening to Jesus teach. They had come from every village in Galilee and Judea and from Jerusalem.

God had given Jesus the power to heal the sick, and some people came carrying a crippled man on a mat. They tried to take him inside the house and put him in front of Jesus. But because of the crowd, they could not get him to Jesus. So they went up on the roof, where they removed some tiles and let the mat down in the middle of the room.

When Jesus saw how much faith they had, he said to the crippled man, "My friend, your sins are forgiven."

The Pharisees and the experts began arguing, "Jesus must think he is God! Only God can forgive sins."

Jesus knew what they were thinking, and he said, "Why are you thinking that? Is it easier for me to tell this crippled man that his sins are forgiven or to tell him to get up and walk? But now you will see that the Son of Man has the right to forgive sins here on earth." Jesus then said to the man, "Get up! Pick up your mat and walk home."

At once the man stood up in front of everyone. He picked up his mat and went home, giving thanks to God. Everyone was amazed and praised God. What they saw surprised them, and they said, "We have seen a great miracle today!" (See also Mark 2:1-12; Matt. 9:1-8)

 Focus on the Scripture

Here stands Jesus in the midst of a rare teaching opportunity. Pharisees and experts in the law of Moses had come from all over Palestine, from every village, to meet and to hear Jesus. The building was bulging with attentive people. Then came an abrupt interruption. Not being able to get in the door, some men got up on the roof, removed a number of roof tiles, and lowered their paralyzed friend into Jesus' presence. Jesus quickly sensed what was happening. Time to stop teaching and start healing. Obviously Jesus was impressed with the initiative, the boldness, the loyalty of these men on behalf of their crippled comrade. No obstacle could turn them back: the jammed doorway, the difficult entry from the roof, or the negative remarks they expected to receive from the religious leaders who had come to hear Jesus teach.

The friends' persistence was rewarded. Luke 5:20 has become the foundational biblical passage for everyone who has ever been motivated to bring friends to Jesus, either literally or by way of intercession. Note that these faith-full friends do not say a word. The man on the mat does not say a word. Perhaps this story illustrates that sincerity of heart and body language are effective ways to pray for others.

This is not the only healing incident in which Jesus combines forgiveness of sin with physical and spiritual healing. Does this connection imply that personal sins cause our personal sicknesses? Sometimes, yes. Sometimes, no. Biblical teachings, as well as current research, clearly indicate that unconfessed sin and unresolved personal guilt can produce an overload of stress and distress, thereby generating a negative impact on one's state of health. This could well be the reason that James 5:14-16 instructs us to confess our sins to one another before we have compassionate Christians pray for our healing.

The unhealthy fallout of our sins can be just as emotionally and spiritually paralyzing as physical paralysis. The unnamed, unspoken, unhealthy man on the mat received a double blessing. His sins were forgiven and his legs walked again. He went home praising God. The critical Pharisees put away their intellectual arguments and their skepticism. This healing action by Jesus spoke louder than any teaching on the subject. The result? The Pharisees also praised God and affirmed this miraculous moment in their lives.

A Reading to Think About

BY MAXIE DUNNAM

In intercession we are united with the entire family of God because we are investing ourselves in the realization of God's reign throughout the universe. Praying in the name of Jesus, we seek for ourselves, our loved ones, and others for whom we have special concern, the gift of God to all [God's] children. So we press for further meaning to praying in the name of Jesus.

In the Bible *names* signify the meaning of character. Names of persons were believed to bear descriptive significance. To know a person's name was more than simply being able to address that person properly.

Praying in the name of Jesus, then, means praying in the powerful love of Jesus, because love was the supreme quality of his whole life.[21]

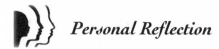 *Personal Reflection*

What is God saying to you in this story?

1. Carefully read and reread the scripture passage. Write down any thoughts, ideas, and questions that may come to you. Do not hurry.

2. Name the specific illness or problem in this story and list all factors that seemed to work together for healing.

3. Ponder the connection between sin and sickness. List types of abusive, sinful behavior that could lead to sickness.

4. For whom are you praying today? As you bring these loved ones and strangers into the healing light and love of Jesus are you faith-full and persistent? What are some obstacles you confront—being too busy, too tired, too discouraged, too worried, too overwhelmed?

5. A United Methodist bishop recovering from eye surgery said to his caring, compassionate Christian friends, "Since I am having difficulty praying as I would like to pray, let me borrow your prayers." Consider this concept of intercessory prayer as lending your prayers, your faith, and your trust in God to other children of God.

Caring Prayer for Others

Carefully review your intercessory prayer list. Then select one person for a time of concentrated, loving, thankful prayer. After you have prayed, be still and listen. Then ask God, Is there something else I could do for this child of God?

Resting in God's Presence

Now put aside your personal agenda and simply relax, basking in the warmth and healing light of God's love.

Go forth from this special place knowing that the grace and peace of Christ go with you!

9

ABSENTEE HEALING

Centering Prayer

O Lord, my Lord, even though I do not deserve all that you do for me, I come to you now, knowing that my worth in your sight does not depend on my good deeds but rather on your good grace. Amen.

Holy Scripture

LUKE 7:1-10

After Jesus had finished teaching the people, he went to Capernaum. In that town an army officer's servant was sick and about to die. The officer liked this servant very much. And when he heard about Jesus, he sent some Jewish leaders to ask him to come and heal the servant.

The leaders went to Jesus and begged him to do something. They said, "This man deserves your help! He loves our nation and even built us a meeting place." So Jesus went with them.

When Jesus wasn't far from the house, the officer sent some friends to tell him, "Lord, don't go to any trouble for me! I am not good enough for you to come into my house. And I am certainly not worthy to come to you. Just say the word, and my servant will get well. I have officers who give orders to me, and I have soldiers who take orders from me. I can say to one of them, 'Go!' and he goes. I can say to another, 'Come!' and he comes. I can say to my servant, 'Do this!' and he will do it."

When Jesus heard this, he was so surprised that he turned and said to the crowd following him, "In all of Israel I've never found anyone with this much faith!" The officer's friends returned and found the servant well. (See also Matt. 8:5-13.)

 Focus on the Scripture

A casual reading of this healing story reminds us of the account of Jesus' curing the nobleman's son in John 4:46-53 (see meditation 22, "Gradual Improvement"). In both stories Jesus does not feel a house call is necessary to bring restored health. After a more studied reading and personal reflection, you will notice significant differences and gain additional insights about absentee healing.

The primary character in Luke's story is an army officer, a centurion in the Roman military occupational forces. A centurion commanded one hundred soldiers. Centurions, the steady, stable, reliable backbone of the Roman army, rightly earned the reputation of being well trained, disciplined, and highly respected. It is not coincidental that whenever the New Testament records a centurion's behavior, the language is complimentary.

The army officer in Luke 7:1-10 is exemplary in every way, including his spiritual understandings. The story presents the problem as the centurion's goal of getting Jesus to heal his deathly ill servant, even though the officer was a Gentile and Jesus, a Jew. Social and religious protocols prohibited the two from entering the privacy of each other's home.

Notice how the centurion circumvented this obstacle. He had his Jewish friends seek out Jesus on his behalf. They explained the situation, adding, "This man deserves your help! He loves our nation and even built us a meeting place" (Luke 7:4-5). It almost seems as though they were bargaining with Jesus: Heal this man's servant in exchange for his good deeds. Never known for following strict protocol, Jesus told them to lead on.

When the centurion learned that Jesus was on the way to his house, he sent his Jewish friends to intercept Jesus a second time with words that totally surprised and amazed everyone, especially Jesus.

The centurion, a man of considerable authority, recognized the higher authority of Jesus and the power of the spoken word. His message to Jesus has since become the genuine prayer of untold millions who recognize their spiritual poverty in the presence of spiritual authority and power: "Lord, do not trouble yourself, for I am not worthy to have you come under my roof. . . . But only speak the word, and let my servant be healed" (Luke 7:6-7, NRSV). Later all discovered to their joy that the servant was indeed healed that very hour. Then Jesus responded in a most remarkable way to the centurion's humbleness: "I tell you, not even in Israel have I found such faith" (Luke 7:9, NRSV).

A Reading to Think About

BY WILLIAM BARCLAY

So Jesus spoke the word and the servant of the centurion was healed. Not so very long ago this would have been a miracle at which the minds of most people would have staggered. It is not so very difficult to think of Jesus healing when he and the sufferer were in actual contact; but to think of Jesus healing at a distance, healing with a word a man he had never seen and never touched, seemed a thing almost, if not completely, beyond belief. But the strange thing is that science itself has come to see that there are forces which are working in a way which is still mysterious, but which is undeniable.

Again and again [people] have been confronted by a power which does not travel by the ordinary contacts and the ordinary routes and the ordinary channels.[22]

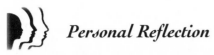 *Personal Reflection*

What is God saying to you in this story?

1. Carefully read and reread the scripture passage. Write down any thoughts, ideas, and questions that may come to you. Do not hurry.

2. Name the specific illness or problem in this story and list all factors that seemed to work together for healing.

3. Try to put yourself into this story by projecting yourself into the mind of Jesus. Record some possible silent thoughts Jesus may have had in response to these comments:

    Luke 7:4-5

    Luke 7:6-7

    Luke 7:8

4. Have you ever bargained with God for special favors? Have you ever intentionally mentioned your latest good deeds in an attempt to focus God's attention on your situation? Our personal worth in God's sight does not depend on our good deeds. Express your heartfelt gratitude for God's grace that not only forgives a multitude of personal sins but also covers unworthiness.

5. Unlike Jesus, whose loving compassion knew no racial or social boundaries, sometimes we have difficulty praying for and accepting anyone who is different from us. The healing of the centurion's servant dramatically informs us that God's grace, healing, and wholeness encircle everyone. Name those you have excluded, and ask your compassionate Savior to help you to be more inclusive.

Caring Prayer for Others

Knowing that absentee healing is entirely possible, pray more boldly and with active, anticipatory faith for those whom God lays on your heart just now.

Resting in God's Presence

Now put aside your personal agenda and simply relax, basking in the warmth and healing light of God's love.

Go forth from this special place knowing that the grace and peace of Christ go with you!

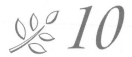 # 10

STRETCH OUT YOUR HAND

Centering Prayer

Lord Jesus Christ, I come to you yearning for a new beginning. Reveal yourself to me in this hour; restore and renew my life and bind me once again to yourself. Amen.[23]

Holy Scripture

MARK 3:1-6

The next time that Jesus went into the meeting place, a man with a crippled hand was there. The Pharisees wanted to accuse Jesus of doing something wrong, and they kept watching to see if Jesus would heal him on the Sabbath.

Jesus told the man to stand up where everyone could see him. Then he asked, "On the Sabbath should we do good deeds or evil deeds? Should we save someone's life or destroy it?" But no one said a word.

Jesus was angry as he looked around at the people. Yet he felt sorry for them because they were so stubborn. Then he told the man, "Stretch out your hand." He did, and his bad hand was healed.

The Pharisees left. And right away they started making plans with Herod's followers to kill Jesus. (See also Luke 6:6-11 and Matt. 12:9-14.)

Focus on the Scripture

As always, the Gospel writer packs a lot into a small package. Here in this brief account is the ongoing controversy over strict Sabbath observances, the amazing healing of a man's severely crippled hand, and the plot to eliminate Jesus. As was his custom, Jesus went to the local synagogue (Jewish meeting place) to teach on the Sabbath (traditional time frame is sundown Friday to sundown Saturday).

Prior to this story, according to Mark's Gospel, Jesus had just had an argument with the Pharisees over his disciples' picking grain to eat on the Sabbath. Jesus responded to the Pharisees with words that were not well received: "People were not made for the good of the Sabbath. The Sabbath was made for the good of people" (Mark 2:27).

Now the stage was set. The Pharisees had reason to see if Jesus would do anything wrong that could lead to his arrest. Jesus knew that by healing on the Sabbath he broke the rules, but he chose to follow a higher rule: people first, Sabbath regulations second. So Jesus invited the man to stand up and to stretch out his hand. The man did not speak, but he did what Jesus asked. Keep in mind that this man could have responded differently. He could have said to Jesus, "Thanks, but no thanks," and left the synagogue. Jesus could have come over to the man and performed the healing without asking him to do anything. But Jesus, respecting the man's dignity and free will, requested his cooperation and participation in the healing process.

Notice a strange thing. Unlike most healing stories, this one includes no mention of rejoicing, gratitude, or praise when the once-withered hand is restored to full function. We can well imagine that the healed man rejoiced; however, we do not have to guess about Jesus' feelings. "Jesus was angry as he looked around at the people. Yet he felt sorry for them because they were so stubborn" (Mark 3:5). They just did not get it that day.

The ending of this story reveals that early in Jesus' public ministry, members of the opposition strategized in making definite plans to destroy him, God's anointed Son, the Messiah. Although doing good for others is often rewarded, doing good can also get one into trouble.

A Reading to Think About

BY TILDA NORBERG AND ROBERT D. WEBBER

The words of Jesus echo through the centuries: "Stretch out your hand." Imagine Jesus saying that to you. Perhaps you can hear in these words an invitation to step out in faith—to let your intellect explore new pathways and allow yourself experiences that might shape your faith in a new way. Maybe you too are being asked to act in faith for your own healing.

Or perhaps you can hear Jesus inviting you to stretch out your hand in compassion to others who need healing. If you have never put your hands on another who is hurting, never prayed for healing, this may indeed be a "stretch" for you.[24]

 Personal Reflection

What is God saying to you in this story?

1. Carefully read and reread the scripture passage. Write down any thoughts, ideas, and questions that may come to you. Do not hurry.

2. Where do you find faith present in this healing story? Given the man's cooperation with Jesus' instructions (he stood up, became the center of attention, and he stretched out his

crippled hand), we could say that he had faith in Jesus to heal him. Could we conclude not only that Jesus had faith in God to provide the healing power but also that Jesus had faith in the man to respond in a positive manner? Meditate on that thought.

3. Have you ever heard or felt Jesus inviting you to come to him simply because Jesus has faith in you to respond? Perhaps faith is a two-way street. We have faith in Jesus, and Jesus has faith in us. Record your thoughts.

4. Think about the location of this healing story that took place in a synagogue, where Judaism's faithful gather for teaching, worship, and fellowship. Those who follow Christ gather in churches for teaching, worship, and fellowship. Have you ever been healed in a church setting? Whenever and wherever the body of Christ gathers, the Risen, Living Lord of the church is present to heal us in body, mind, spirit, and in all our relationships. Pause here to express your gratitude for Christ's healing ministry. The next time you worship, especially at Holy Communion, affirm the healing presence of Christ and ask him to make whole any area of your life that is unhealthy. Write down your personal health needs and lift them to Christ in prayer right now.

5. Have you ever gotten into trouble because you did something good for someone? Goodness is sometimes rewarded with unkind criticism. Good deeds, however well intended,

are not always received with appreciation. This healing story teaches us that Jesus did not do good for others in order to receive adoration and praise.

Reflect on this thought: Jesus' interior motive was to help others simply because they needed help. Always his goal was to improve the human condition, to give God the glory, and not to worry about the fallout. If your good deeds are driven by different motives, then you will not be able to stand up when you are put down. Examine your personal motives for helping others. Write down any thoughts.

Caring Prayer for Others

Pray by name for persons who do not seem to be open and receptive to Jesus Christ, whose hope, help, and healing could become a reality with their cooperation.

Resting in God's Presence

Now put aside your personal agenda and simply relax, basking in the warmth and healing light of God's love.

Go forth from this special place knowing that the grace and peace of Christ go with you!

11

DOES FAITH HEAL?

Centering Prayer

I come now in faith and by faith in you, O Christ, knowing that apart from you, I am not complete or whole. I know and trust that you truly care about everything going on in my life. Amen.

Holy Scripture

LUKE 8:43-48

In the crowd was a woman who had been bleeding for twelve years. She had spent everything she had on doctors, but none of them could make her well.

As soon as she came up behind Jesus and barely touched his clothes, her bleeding stopped.

"Who touched me?" Jesus asked.

While everyone was denying it, Peter said, "Master, people are crowding all around and pushing you from every side."

But Jesus answered, "Someone touched me, because I felt power going out from me." The woman knew that she could not hide, so she came trembling and knelt down in front of Jesus. She told everyone why she had touched him and that she had been healed right away.

Jesus said to the woman, "You are now well because of your faith. May God give you peace!" (See also Mark 5:25-34 and Matt. 9:20-22.)

Focus on the Scripture

Here is a portrait of a desperate woman. After years of seeking medical help for her health problem, she continued to suffer physically and emotionally. In first-century Jewish culture, no one would touch or even go near a woman who was hemorrhaging. Twelve years is a long time to be a social outcast. When she heard that Jesus was coming her way, this discouraged, despondent woman decided to take a great risk by getting close enough to Jesus simply to touch his clothing. When she did this she got immediate results. Not only did her bleeding stop, but the super-sensitive Jesus also stopped to give her his undivided attention when he felt power going out from his body. Sensing that she was healed, the woman's timidity shifted to boldness in telling the crowd what had happened and in giving Jesus the credit. You can well imagine that this nameless woman never, ever forgot Jesus' parting words to her, "You are now well because of your faith. May God give you peace."

This marvelous story raises many questions for the health-conscious reader:

- How much can we depend on the medical profession for our total health care?

- What is the role of faith in the healing process?

- Do some people have more faith in their health-care insurance than they do in the Healing Christ?

- Does Christ continue to heal people today?

Let us affirm and thank God for all who dedicate themselves to the health-care professions. Without doubt God uses medical means to heal every day. However, because of our God-given spirituality, we need to use the best medical care *and* the best spiritual care. The woman in the story had tried the medical options of her day and now actively sought spiritual help.

Current research points to the most influential factor in determining our overall health: our personal lifestyle, that is, our personal habits, our personal beliefs and values. Doctors do not cure us. Doctors work to create an environment within our bodies and minds that helps to restore balance and activate the God-given healing agents within us. As one doctor responded to a young couple's request to have prayer with their newborn baby whose heart was not functioning properly, "I think you should [pray]. I'm only the helper."[25]

A Reading to Think About

BY DALE A. MATTHEWS, M.D.

The research findings made me a confirmed believer in the widespread benefits of the remarkable catalyst for health called "the faith factor."[26]

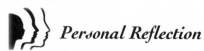 *Personal Reflection*

What is God saying to you in this story?

1. Carefully read and reread the scripture passage. Write down any thoughts, ideas, and questions that may come to you. Do not hurry.

2. Name the specific illness or problem in this story and list all factors that seemed to work together for healing.

3. On a scale of 1 to 10, with 10 being the highest value, what ranking would you give your faith in Christ's ability to heal you? Record your thoughts about combining the best medical care and the best spiritual care when you or a loved one becomes ill.

4. Visualization Prayer: Read these guidelines and then close your eyes. Imagine you are that woman in the story with a problem that will not go away. Name your dilemma. It may be physical, spiritual, emotional, or a relationship issue. Knowing that Jesus cares deeply about your total life situation, make your way into his presence. In faith and trust, reach out to him. When Jesus focuses his attention on you, what do you say? What does he say to you? Listen. Listen. Listen. Open your eyes and record your feelings and thoughts.

5. Offer a sincere prayer of thanksgiving not only for this marvelous story in the Gospels but also for the Healing Christ in your life this very moment. Receive his words of assurance: "My daughter, my son, your faith has made you well. Your faith has made a positive difference in your life. Your faith has saved you. Now go in peace. Take care of yourself. Stay healthy."

Caring Prayer for Others

Name friends and family members who are dealing with chronic, ongoing health problems. Lift them lovingly with thanksgiving into the healing light of Christ.

Resting in God's Presence

Now put aside your personal agenda and simply relax, basking in the warmth and healing light of God's love.

Go forth from this special place knowing that the grace and peace of Christ go with you!

12

DON'T WORRY! HAVE FAITH!

Centering Prayer

As a young child yearns to be in the caring, understanding, protective presence of parents, so I come to you, O God, my heavenly Father. Help me to relax, to feel your love, and to hear your word. Amen.

Holy Scripture

LUKE 8:40-42, 49-56

Everyone had been waiting for Jesus, and when he came back, a crowd was there to welcome him. Just then the man in charge of the Jewish meeting place came and knelt down in front of Jesus. His name was Jairus, and he begged Jesus to come to his home because his twelve-year-old child was dying. She was his only daughter.

While Jesus was on his way, people were crowding all around him. . . .

While Jesus was speaking, someone came from Jairus' home and said, "Your daughter has died! Why bother the teacher anymore?"

When Jesus heard this, he told Jairus, "Don't worry! Have faith, and your daughter will get well." Jesus went into the house, but he did not let anyone else go with him, except Peter, John, James, and the girl's father and mother. Everyone was crying and weeping for the girl. But Jesus said, "The child isn't. She is just asleep." The people laughed at him because they knew she was dead.

Jesus took hold of the girl's hand and said, "Child, get up!" She came back to life and got right up. Jesus told them to give her something to eat. Her parents were surprised, but Jesus ordered them not to tell anyone what had happened. (See also Mark 5:21-24, 35-43 and Matt. 9:18-19, 23-26.)

Focus on the Scripture

We are grateful to the Gospel author Luke, as well as to Mark and Matthew, for including this unusual healing story in their written narratives about Jesus. Not only does this scripture demonstrate Jesus' tender compassion for children but it shows again his ability to handle interruptions. Actually, if you read this passage in context (Luke 8:40-56), you have a well-crafted story within a story, with some notable similarities:

- Here are two female characters with health problems: a woman who has been sick for twelve years and a twelve-year-old girl.

- Both are nameless; both are referred to as "daughter."

- Each one is critically ill.

The connecting link to these intertwined stories is that both the desperate father and the despondent woman turn to Jesus in total, complete, no-doubt-about-it faith.

Jesus commends the woman for her witness to her healing and for her faith. The young girl, however, does not speak. We know nothing about her faith, but we do know that her father, Jairus, truly has faith in Jesus to heal. When you or your loved ones are critically ill, perhaps in a coma or in an irrational state of mind, the genuine faith of others operating and praying on your behalf can be the catalyst, the plus factor, in the healing process.

When the bearer of bad news announced that Jairus's daughter had died and Jairus should not bother the famous rabbi, Jesus countered, "She is not dead. She is asleep." The key to her healing, however, is in Jesus' bold encouragement to Jairus, "Don't worry! Have faith, and your daughter will get well" (8:50). The father, a leading citizen in the Jewish community, took a great risk simply by coming to Jesus publicly. However, the rewards of faith in Jesus always outweigh the risks we take for Jesus.

A Reading to Think About

BY DONALD BARTOW

It is important to realize that faith is a vital part of the healing process. It is important that you believe the Lord wants you to be whole.

It is even of greater importance for you to believe He is able to make you whole.[27]

Personal Reflection

 What is God saying to you in this story?

1. Carefully read and reread the scripture passage. Write down any thoughts, ideas, and questions that may come to you. Do not hurry.

2. Name the specific illness or problem in this story and list all factors that seemed to work together for healing.

3. Did you notice this significant piece of information in Luke 8:42: "She was his only daughter"? Jairus may or may not have had sons. The girl may have been his only child. Desperate parents do desperate things when their children are at the point of death. Put yourself in this story. If your only child were critically ill, what would you do?

4. As you ponder the role of faith in the healing process, reflect on this key scripture passage: "Now faith is the assurance of things hoped for, the conviction of things not seen. . . . And without faith it is impossible to please God, for whoever would approach him must believe that he exists and that he rewards those who seek him" (Heb. 11:1, 6 NRSV).

5. Pray for God to give you a faith in Christ to live by and to die by, whatever the circumstances and situations you may face.

Caring Prayer for Others

Knowing that Jesus has a special place in his heart for all children, lift in prayer by name several children in your world.

Resting in God's Presence

Now put aside your personal agenda and simply relax, basking in the warmth and healing of God's love.

Go forth from this special place knowing that the grace and peace of Christ go with you!

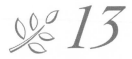 # *13*

EVIL CONFRONTED

Centering Prayer

> Create in me a clean heart, O God,
>> and put a new and right spirit within me.
> Do not cast me away from your presence,
>> and do not take your holy spirit from me.
> Restore to me the joy of your salvation,
>> and sustain in me a willing spirit (Ps. 51:10-12, NRSV).

Holy Scripture

MARK 1:21-28

Jesus and his disciples went to the town of Capernaum. Then on the next Sabbath he went into the Jewish meeting place and started teaching. Everyone was amazed at his teaching. He taught with authority, and not like the teachers of the Law of Moses. Suddenly a man with an evil spirit in him entered the meeting place and yelled, "Jesus from Nazareth, what do you want with us? Have you come to destroy us? I know who you are! You are God's Holy One."

Jesus told the evil spirit, "Be quiet and come out of the man!" The spirit shook him. Then it gave a loud shout and left.

Everyone was completely surprised and kept saying to each other, "What is this? It must be some new kind of powerful teaching! Even the evil spirits obey him." News about Jesus quickly spread all over Galilee. (See also Luke 4:31-37.)

Focus on the Scripture

In this story, as in several healing stories in the Gospel records, Jesus openly, boldly, and confidently confronts evil in the form of demons and spirits that torment and confuse. These particular stories raise several issues for contemporary readers. Whereas first-century citizens easily believed in the reality of evil forces at loose in the world, many readers in the twenty-first century either skip lightly over the evil-spirit passages in the New Testament or dismiss them as hardly more than the early church trying to explain what we call "mental illness." Indeed the modern medical profession could well diagnose as epilepsy the erratic behavior people in biblical times believed to be demon possession.

Anyone thought to have an evil spirit was considered "unclean" and not allowed to eat or to worship with other people in the Jewish meeting places. This cultural taboo explains the initial amazement of the assembled congregation over the authority with which Jesus taught and their complete astonishment at Jesus' ability to command respect and obedience from evil spirits.

When it comes to dealing with the reality of evil in today's world, people were forced to acknowledge the demonic nature of the devastating actions on September 11, 2001, when terrorist attacks brought horrific suffering and tragedy. We can no longer ignore evil, making it an unmentionable subject from the pulpit, in classrooms, and in daily conversations. Nor should we overreact and blame evil spirits for every problem imaginable. Taking our cue from Jesus, we can believe in the spiritual realm and in the kingdom of God, where God is in charge of everyone and everything. However, God's kingdom has not come fully on earth as it is in heaven, where God supremely reigns. For this reason, Jesus cautioned all who claim him as Lord and Savior that Satan (sometimes called the devil or the evil one) will do whatever is required to oppose God's plans. Notice the word *evil* is *live* spelled backward. The opposite of life, goodness, and eternal values is always evil. This is why Jesus taught us in his model prayer to seek God's powerful assistance in dealing with evil by praying the petition "Deliver us from evil" (Matt. 6:13, KJV).

A Reading to Think About

BY L. DAVID MITCHELL

The devil incites men, women and children to rebel against God and all that is good, and to serve the cause of self and sin. Demonic powers lust to corrupt people in their imagination. John Wesley once warned that it is easier for the devil to put a picture into the mind of a man than it is for one man to whisper into the ear of another. The enemy wants to devour humans by playing upon their natural appetites and needs. Every existing situation and relationship, every potentiality can be his target. The evil-one is, simultaneously, both gross and obvious (to discerning Christians) and subtly clever in his battle for human souls.

This is the original spiritual conflict that began in the Garden of Eden and will continue until the return of Christ. Meanwhile, "We have the right man on our side," as Luther's hymn melodiously puts it, Christ himself. He will never leave us or forsake us. In constant faithfulness, from moment to moment, he gives gracious comfort, encouragement, strength and spiritual authority to those who have been reborn by the Holy Spirit.[28]

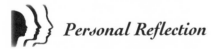 *Personal Reflection*

What is God saying to you in this story?

1. Carefully read and reread the scripture passage. Write down any thoughts, ideas, and questions that may come to you. Do not hurry.

2. Name the specific illness or problem in this story and list all factors that seemed to work together for healing.

3. Try to imagine that you are there, actually present that day in the synagogue at Capernaum. You are meeting Jesus of Nazareth for the first time. You are in that congregation listening and observing everything. How would you react

to the authority in the teachings of Jesus?

to the interruption by the out-of-control man who came into the room and started yelling at Jesus?

to the way Jesus dealt with the man and with the apparent evil spirits?

to Jesus' demonstration of authority over evil, which gave added authenticity to his teachings?

4. Consider the man calmed down and delivered from evil. If you had been that man, what would you have felt, thought, done, or said to Jesus?

5. What is your personal understanding of evil? If you have not given serious thought to the reality of evil, now is the time to begin. Write down your unanswered questions.

Then, without rushing, pray silently or aloud the prayer Jesus taught his disciples: "Our Father in heaven, hallowed be your name, your kingdom come, your will be done, on earth as in heaven. Give us today our daily bread. Forgive us our sins as we forgive those who sin against us. Save us from the time of trial and deliver us from evil. For the kingdom, the power, and the glory are yours now and forever. Amen."[29]

Caring Prayer for Others

Pray by name for persons you know who are excluded and not allowed to enter into certain social or community activities because they seem to be different.

Resting in God's Presence

Now put aside your personal agenda and simply relax, basking in the warmth and healing light of God's love.

Go forth from this special place knowing that the grace and peace of Christ go with you!

14

EVIL IS REAL

Centering Prayer

O God, my Creator and Protector, I now close the door of my spirit to all and to everything except the loving, forgiving, healing, empowering Spirit of Christ. Amen.

Holy Scripture

LUKE 8:26-39

Jesus and his disciples sailed across Lake Galilee and came to shore near the town of Gerasa. As Jesus was getting out of the boat, he was met by a man from that town. The man had demons in him. He had gone naked for a long time and no longer lived in a house, but in the graveyard.

The man saw Jesus and screamed. He knelt down in front of him and shouted, "Jesus, Son of God in heaven, what do you want with me? I beg you not to torture me!" He said this because Jesus had already told the evil spirit to go out of him.

The man had often been attacked by the demon. And even though he had been bound with chains and leg irons and kept under guard, he smashed whatever bound him. Then the demon would force him out into lonely places.

Jesus asked the man, "What is your name?"

He answered, "My name is Lots." He said this because there were "lots" of demons in him. They begged Jesus not to send them to the deep pit, where they would be punished.

A large herd of pigs was feeding there on the hillside. So the demons begged Jesus to let them go into the pigs, and Jesus let them go. Then the demons left the man and went into the pigs. The whole herd rushed down the steep bank into the lake and drowned.

When the men taking care of the pigs saw this, they ran to spread the news in the town and on the farms. The people went out to see what had happened, and when they came to Jesus, they also found the man. The demons had gone out of him, and he was sitting there at the feet of Jesus. He had clothes on and was in his right mind. But the people were terrified.

Then all who had seen the man healed told about it. Everyone from around Gerasa begged Jesus to leave, because they were so frightened.

When Jesus got into the boat to start back, the man who had been healed begged to go with him. But Jesus sent him off and said, "Go back home and tell everyone how much God has done for you." The man then went all over town, telling everything that Jesus had done for him. (See also Mark 5:1-20 and Matt. 8:28-34.)

 Focus on the Scripture

The often-prayed petition in the Lord's Prayer "Deliver us from evil" alerts us not only to the reality of evil in our world but also to the need of a power greater than our own to rescue and protect us from active evil forces. The tormented and deranged man in this story was possessed by several demons or evil spirits who had taken up residence in his body and mind. Because he could not control these demons, he could not control his behavior. Consequently he was forced to live outside the town, apart from other human beings. Popular belief held that demons and evil spirits lived in graveyards. The only acceptable habitat for him, therefore, was the local cemetery.

When Jesus arrived on that desolate scene, he knew that rational counseling, a loving physical touch, or a prayer for healing would be ineffective. So he engaged in what is now called an exorcism, speaking directly not to the distraught man but to the demons, ordering them to get out of him. After a bit of protesting, the demons left the man, entered a herd of pigs, and drowned in the lake. Although this method of curing the man is difficult for us to understand, the result was awesome. When the local residents came to the cemetery to find out what had happened to the pigs, they discovered the former demoniac "sitting there at the feet of Jesus. He had clothes on and was in his right mind" (Luke 8:35).

Were the curious folks pleased and happy for this total reversal in the man's personality? Just the opposite. Not knowing how to deal with the healed man or with the healer, they were terrified and ordered Jesus to leave immediately. The man, anticipating more confrontation from his neighbors, begged Jesus to take him along. Instead Jesus sent the cured man home to tell everyone what God had done for him.

Total possession of a human being by evil is rare, and exorcisms are not common; nor were they in biblical times. Scriptures and human experience witness not so much to persons' being completely possessed but being temporarily oppressed by evil forces. Evil becomes influential in our lives only when our personal sins and human weaknesses allow it.

Unlike total possession by evil, being oppressed is a impermanent, passing situation. Likewise, at times we may become obsessed or attracted to certain evil influences when we give in to personal temptations. Obsession with evil may become addictive, but it can be cured and eliminated with appropriate therapy. Jesus had the spiritual sensitivity to distinguish between oppression, obsession, and possession. The Holy Spirit's gift of discernment of spirits is crucial for those Christians engaged in deliverance ministries.

A Reading to Think About

BY FRANCIS MACNUTT

We cannot really understand [evil] unless we come to grips with certain realities:

1. Evil is something we cannot overcome by simple human good will and teaching. Evil is, at its root, demonic and too great for us to overcome.
2. It is for this purpose that Jesus came: to overcome evil.
3. Evil cannot be overcome just through teaching ethical values, but by the power of God, which is given to us by the Holy Spirit.
4. Through prayer—prayer for healing and prayer for deliverance—we become channels for Jesus to heal and to free people (as well as institutions and societies) from the evil that weighs them down.

Jesus' ministry of deliverance is central to an understanding of the Gospel:

"The reason the Son of God appeared was to destroy the devil's work" (1 John 3:8).[30]

 Personal Reflection

What is God saying to you in this story?

1. Carefully read and reread the scripture passage. Write down any thoughts, ideas, and questions that may come to you. Do not hurry.

2. Name the specific illness or problem in this story and list all factors that seemed to work together for healing.

3. Defining evil as the opposite of life, goodness, and eternal values, make a list of people, current events, and situations that seem to illustrate the continuing presence and negative impact of evil in today's world.

4. In addition to calling on the power, protection, and deliverance of Christ, what else can you do to protect yourself and your loved ones from evil influences?

5. The healing process includes telling others (witnessing) what the Lord has done for you, as Jesus instructed the man to do in the story. When was the last time you gave God the credit for something good that happened in your life? Have you shared this news with others?

Caring Prayer for Others

Lift in prayer those persons you know who may be dealing with oppression, confusion, and at times out-of-control evil influences in their lives. Ask Christ to deliver, heal, and protect them.

Resting in God's Presence

Now put aside your personal agenda and simply relax, basking in the warmth and healing light of God's love.

Go forth from this special place knowing that the grace and peace of Christ go with you!

15

PROTECTION FROM EVIL

Centering Prayer

As I come to you right now, God of all blessings and goodness, I anticipate my spirit's being renewed by the Spirit of Christ, my mind's being restored by the mind of Christ, my body's being healed by the power of Christ, and my personal relationships' being enhanced, blessed, and bonded by the love of Christ. Amen.

Holy Scripture

MATTHEW 12:22-28

Some people brought to Jesus a man who was blind and could not talk because he had a demon in him. Jesus healed the man, and then he was able to talk and see. The crowds were so amazed that they asked, "Could Jesus be the Son of David?"

When the Pharisees heard this, they said, "He forces out demons by the power of Beelzebul, the ruler of the demons!"

Jesus knew what they were thinking, and he said to them:

> Any kingdom where people fight each other will end up ruined. And a town or family that fights will soon destroy itself. So if Satan fights against himself, how can his kingdom last? If I use the power of Beelzebul to force out demons, whose power do your own followers use to force them out? Your followers are the ones who will judge you. But when I

force out demons by the power of God's Spirit, it proves that God's kingdom has already come to you.

(See also Mark 3:20-30 and Luke 11:14-20.)

 ## *Focus on the Scripture*

Do not confuse this healing story with the one in Mark 7:31-37 about the man who was deaf and had a speech impairment (see meditation 20, "The Sensitivity of Jesus").

Jesus exhibited complete sensitivity to the unique needs of each individual's situation. Jesus did not assume that every illness and impaired condition was demon-instigated or a case of demon possession. According to Matthew 12:22, some people brought this man to Jesus because they believed an evil spirit was causing the blindness and speech disability. Matthew does not tell us what method Jesus used in restoring this man's vision and ability to talk. Because Jesus was no cookie-cutter–type healer, he used a variety of ways to help others—a good lesson for those of us who feel led to engage in healing ministry.

Although the details of this story differ in the three accounts by Matthew, Mark, and Luke, all three record the conversation between Jesus and certain persons in the crowd who were questioning not so much his ability but rather his authority in casting out demons, accusing Jesus of using the power of Beelzebul, ruler of demons. However, they cannot "outargue" Jesus, who reinforces his authority as coming directly from God. God absolutely opposes evil in every form, and God's kingdom has the upper hand.

A Reading to Think About

BY ALBERT E. DAY

The kingdom of God has a tremendous social significance. But its impact upon society awaits its realization in the lives of individuals.

"Thy kingdom come, *beginning with me.*" It must begin here, or it cannot operate in the social order. Its agents are not "principalities and powers" operating from the unseen; but persons operating on the scene, infusing a new spirit, creating new institutions, writing new laws, inaugurating a new era. It came near in Jesus: "The kingdom of God has come upon you" (Luke 11:20, RSV). It has been coming ever since where men and women first enthrone God in their own lives.[31]

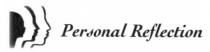 *Personal Reflection*

What is God saying to you in this story?

1. Carefully read and reread the scripture passage. Write down any thoughts, ideas, and questions that may come to you. Do not hurry.

2. Name the specific illness or problem in this story and list all factors that seemed to work together for healing.

3. Because of our God-given free will, neither good nor evil can take root in our lives without our permission or cooperation. The kingdom of God comes into our individual lives when self is dethroned and Christ is enthroned. Who is sitting on the throne of your life today? What are some ways you can let Christ be in charge of your life?

4. We are never "home free" from the evil one's desire to influence our lives. Reflect on this verse: "Discipline yourselves, keep alert. Like a roaring lion your adversary the devil prowls around, looking for someone to devour" (1 Pet. 5:8, NRSV). The best protection from evil is to saturate oneself frequently with God's means of grace: Holy Communion, prayer, time alone with God, Bible reading and study, Christ-centered worship, Christian music, fasting, active church membership, frequent fellowship with other Christians, engaging in deeds of mercy, and an intentional renewal of one's commitment to Christ every day. Which of these means of God's grace do you need most in your life? Develop an action plan for this practice.

5. In this story people bring to Jesus a man who needed help only Jesus could give. Name friends, acquaintances, neighbors, or family members you could invite to your church, Bible study group, Sunday school class, or other Christian gatherings who may not know Jesus personally or who may

not have a church home or who need healing in body, mind, spirit, or in a relationship.

Caring Prayer for Others

Pray for each person you have named in number 5 above. Seek the guidance of the Holy Spirit in knowing what to do next in bringing those individuals to Jesus.

Resting in God's Presence

Now put aside your personal agenda and simply relax, basking in the warmth and healing light of God's love.

Go forth from this special place knowing that the grace and peace of Christ go with you!

16

HOMETOWN REJECTION

Centering Prayer

Heal me, hands of Jesus, and search out all my pain;
  restore my hope, remove my fear, and bring me
    peace again.
. . . .
Fill me, joy of Jesus; anxiety shall cease,
  and heaven's serenity be mine, for Jesus brings me peace![32]

Holy Scripture

MARK 6:1-6

Jesus left and returned to his hometown with his disciples. The next Sabbath he taught in the Jewish meeting place. Many of the people who heard him were amazed and asked, "How can he do all this? Where did he get such wisdom and the power to work these miracles? Isn't he the carpenter, the son of Mary? Aren't James, Joseph, Judas, and Simon his brothers? Don't his sisters still live here in our town?" The people were unhappy because of what he was doing.

But Jesus said, "Prophets are honored by everyone, except the people of their hometown and their relatives and their own family." Jesus could not work any miracles there, except to heal a few sick people by placing his hands on them. He was surprised that the people did not have any faith (See also Matt. 13:53-58 and Luke 4:16-30.)

Focus on the Scripture

Even though this incident in Jesus' boyhood village of Nazareth occurred early in his public ministry, Jesus was already attracting large crowds wherever he went, according to the Gospel writers. Luke's account of Jesus' hometown rejection contrasts sharply with the passage immediately prior: "Jesus returned to Galilee with the power of the Spirit. News about him spread everywhere. He taught in the Jewish meeting places, and everyone praised him" (Luke 4:14-15).

Obviously Jesus was not prepared for the hostile greeting in the Nazareth synagogue. You can feel Jesus' sadness and disappointment. His neighbors questioned everything he did and taught. After all, he was only the son of a carpenter. They knew his brothers and sisters, many of whom still lived in Nazareth. What was so special about Mary's boy now grown up? Their negativity served only to hamper his ministry among them. One of the saddest passages in all the Gospels is Mark 6:5-6: "Jesus could not work any miracles there, except to heal a few sick people by placing his hands on them. He was surprised that the people did not have any faith."

This visit to the Nazareth synagogue essentially failed, and in Mark's Gospel there is no record that Jesus ever entered that synagogue again; instead, he chose other strategies to get his message out to the people. However, even failure can produce positive lessons for those who believe all of life is a learning experience. Jesus discovered that without human cooperation and a trusting faith, his powers were indeed limited. That truth still holds today. Jesus cannot and will not force his goodness, mercy, and love on anyone. Our cooperation and faith in Jesus must blend with God's desire for our health, wholeness, and salvation.

Jesus did not engage in a lengthy discussion, chastising the skeptical citizens of Nazareth. He wisely quoted a known proverb and let it go at that: "Prophets are honored by everyone, except the people of their hometown and their relatives and their own family" (Mark 6:4). This observation by Jesus indicates his ability to analyze a situation, evaluate what is happening, and get on with his life. A lesser prophet might have retired on the spot, but the last line of this story clearly shows us that Jesus' ministry did not depend on high praise, pats on the back, and constant approval. His God-inspired vision transcended petty bickering. So he said his good-byes and got on with his mission. Jesus left Nazareth and "taught in all the neighboring villages" (Mark 6:6).

A Reading to Think About

BY MILDRED THOMAS

When I flick an electric switch and the light appears, I sometimes think of Thomas Edison and his remarkable contribution to the lighting we enjoy. His life-story reveals that what once must have looked like Edison's trials actually contributed to his triumphs. . . .

That dreamer and inventor was a tireless worker, and he was not easily discouraged. When he and his team were experimenting on ways to make his electric bulb last more than a few hours, they worked faithfully for a long time without success. After the sixth early burn-out someone asked him, "Won't you admit you have failed?" Edison replied: "These weren't failures. They were learning experiences."

Edison went on to turn his trials into triumphs. What a difference one's attitude can make![33]

 Personal Reflection

What is God saying to you in this story?

1. Carefully read and reread the scripture passage. Write down any thoughts, ideas, and questions that may come to you. Do not hurry.

2. Because Jesus had a clear understanding of who he was and what his goals were, he never lost his focus when things did not go his way. You are a child of God, loved unconditionally by God. Nothing can separate you from God's mercy and grace given to you every day. Therefore how important is constant approval from others? List your fundamental goals in life. Write down what you value most. Where on your list do you place your personal relationship with God?

3. Put yourself in the mind and heart of Jesus. How do you imagine Jesus felt when the people were unhappy with him in Nazareth that day? How do you deal with personal rejection in your life? How do you handle personal criticisms? What can you learn from Jesus' style of coping with disappointments?

4. Test out this saying for yourself: "All of life is a learning experience." Make a list of ten personal experiences: five negative and five positive. Then ask this question of each one: What are some things I learned from this experience?

5. We frequently hear the saying "Familiarity breeds contempt." Let us revise this thought with a question: Could it be that some Christians are so familiar with Jesus and his teachings that their joy is jaded, their prayer life is boring, and daily expectations of him are almost nonexistent? Be honest! Do you really know Jesus? Try rereading the four Gospels as though you were seeing the words and learning about Jesus for the first time. Ponder deeply your personal relationship with Jesus right now. Then enter into a prayer-conversation with him as your heart and spirit lead you.

Caring Prayer for Others

As you engage in prayer about your personal relationship with Jesus, lift names of family members and friends whose daily walk with Jesus seems to lack vitality. Place them in God's loving hands. Offer prayers of thanksgiving and blessings for each one.

Resting in God's Presence

Now put aside your personal agenda and simply relax, basking in the warmth and healing light of God's love.

Go forth from this special place knowing that the grace and peace of Christ go with you!

17

GO AND TELL

Centering Prayer

O timeless and timely God, I thank you for the gift of time and especially for this time together. May I hear with joy what you say to me and may you receive with understanding what I bring to you. In the name of Christ who redeems the time, I come to you now. Amen.

Holy Scripture

LUKE 7:18-23

John's followers told John everything that was being said about Jesus. So he sent two of them to ask the Lord, "Are you the one we should be looking for? Or must we wait for someone else?"

When these messengers came to Jesus, they said, "John the Baptist sent us to ask, 'Are you the one we should be looking for? Or are we supposed to wait for someone else?'"

At that time Jesus was healing many people who were sick or in pain or were troubled by evil spirits, and he was giving sight to a lot of blind people. Jesus said to the messengers sent by John, "Go and tell John what you have seen and heard. Blind people are now able to see, and the lame can walk. People who have leprosy are being healed, and the deaf can now hear. The dead are raised to life, and the poor are hearing the good news. God will bless everyone who does not reject me because of what I do." (See also Matt. 11:2-6.)

Focus on the Scripture

As we grow older and our lives take turns and twists we had not anticipated, we often question ideas and ideals we thought we had settled forever in our younger years. Jesus' famous cousin called John the Baptizer experienced this kind of questioning. Recall that on the eve of Jesus' going public with his three-year ministry, he purposely went to John and submitted to being baptized by John, whom he highly respected for many reasons. This baptism proved to be a spiritual high point for both Jesus and John. (See the full account in Luke 3:1-22.)

The two men then went their separate ways: John continued to gather disciples, and Jesus recruited his followers. John got into deep trouble with the political authorities by publicly condemning King Herod for a series of unjust, brutal, and deceptive actions. Consequently John was cruelly imprisoned by Herod and cut off from the world. Put yourself in John's place in that jail cell for a moment. Would you not be reviewing the past events of your life? Would you not be questioning God's possible intervention in the chaos and corruption of your world? Would you perhaps have a doubt or two about the authenticity and authority of your cousin Jesus? Could John have been wrong about him?

This is where the story picks up in our focus scripture, Luke 7:18-23. John obviously needed reassurance that Jesus truly was the long-awaited messiah. So John sent two of his disciples to find Jesus and to ask him the question that thinking, questing, spiritually hungry human beings are still asking today: "Are you the one we should be looking for? Or must we wait for someone else?" Notice this question is repeated, a sign of special significance (see Luke 7:20).

Jesus could have responded, "Yes, I am the one." Instead, he instructed John's disciples to go back to John with a litany of signs and wonders that not only would renew John's faith and courage but also would give him the assurance to bear him up no matter what might happen.

"Go and tell John what you have seen and heard. I have given hope to the hopeless: the blind, the lame, the deaf, the lepers, the poor. And, yes, even the dead are raised to new life." If you had been John on the receiving end of this good news, would not your personal hope have been renewed? Actually Jesus was telling John that the prophecy of Isaiah 61:1-2 was being carried out and fulfilled by Jesus. Jesus read this passage in his hometown synagogue when he returned, and he then told the congregation what he intended to do at the beginning of his ministry. (See Luke 4:16-21.)

To paraphrase Jesus' words in Luke 7:22-23, "If you have difficulty believing I am who I say I am, then let my good works speak for themselves. Those of you who still doubt, let my track record settle it for you." Or, as we say today, "Actions speak louder than words." Throughout his brief public career Jesus constantly dealt with people (his own disciples as well as strangers) who questioned whether Jesus was who he said he was. Jesus said, "Have faith in me when I say that the Father is one with me and that I am one with the Father. Or else have faith in me simply because of the things I do" (John 14:11).

A Reading to Think About

BY G. ERNEST THOMAS

For almost two thousand years Christians have accepted Jesus of Nazareth as the perfect reflection of God. They have declared that persons who want to know what God is like may safely look to Jesus. They have made him the author and example of the kind of personal living which has the seal of God upon it.

The challenge of the Christian faith is direct and forceful. It speaks to every individual who really wants to know God. It says: "Why not try the way of Christ?" "Why not accept his picture of God?" "Why not do the things [God] asks?"[34]

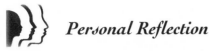 *Personal Reflection*

What is God saying to you in this story?

1. Carefully read and reread the scripture passage. Write down any thoughts, ideas, and questions that may come to you. Do not hurry.

2. Have you ever asked or are you asking now about Jesus: Are you the one we should be looking for, or must we wait for someone else? Jesus answered that question in John 14:6, NRSV: "I am the way, and the truth, and the life." What would you have Jesus do differently or in addition to what he has done already to convince people that he is God's messiah for the whole world?

3. Healing is a process. Sometimes we do experience that amazing, instantaneous miracle cure, but usually we get well by gradual improvement. In either time span, we know, through the healing ministry of Jesus, that God cares about every illness and health problem we face. If you are not 100 percent healthy today, invite God's healing presence, the living

111

Christ, to touch your life, to guide you in your healing process, and to make you well again. What areas of your life need the wholeness and health of Christ?

4. "Go and tell John what you have seen and heard," Jesus said to John's disciples. That is also good counsel for the followers of Jesus today. Record some recent personal illnesses that now are healed. Whom did you thank when you recovered? If you truly believe that God was working with your doctor, your medications, prayer groups, and other kinds of therapy, did you thank God? More importantly, did you go and tell others that God healed you? Witnessing to others not only strengthens your personal faith but also plants seeds of faith and encourages others to place their trust and confidence in God. What are some ways you could "go and tell" your friends at church? (See Pss. 22:22; 35:18; 40:9-10; 149:1.)

5. Have you ever had conversation with someone skeptical about Jesus and critical of Christians? Have you ever met those who said they wanted to believe in Jesus and his teachings but had so many personal questions they simply could not? A wise Christian pastor says to doubting inquirers: "Try Jesus for six months. Read a portion of the four Gospels every day and with God's help try to live out the

teachings of the Bible every day. Pray as you are able, not as you think you should or ought to pray. Let your prayers be as conversation between best friends. God will respect your honesty and will not disappoint you. Come back in six months and let's discuss the matter further. Go in peace!" Record the names of persons you know who indicate a desire to believe in Jesus but cannot for some reason.

Caring Prayer for Others

Begin by thanking God for Jesus, for his life and ministry, and especially for his care and concern for the least, the lost, and the hopeless. Then pray for the Spirit of Jesus, the Risen Christ, to bless, help, and bring hope to those persons you now name out of your own faith, compassion, and love.

Resting in God's Presence

Now put aside your personal agenda and simply relax, basking in the warmth and healing light of God's love.

Go forth from this special place knowing that the grace and peace of Christ go with you!

18

THE FAITHLESS DISCIPLES

Centering Prayer

O God, who gave the name Jesus to your special Son, the name that is above all names, I come to you with many problems, concerns, and challenges in my life. Yet I also come to you with prayer in my heart and praise in my soul anticipating with joy our time together. In Jesus' name. Amen.

Holy Scripture

MATTHEW 17:14-21

Jesus and his disciples returned to the crowd. A man knelt in front of him and said, "Lord, have pity on my son! He has a bad case of epilepsy and often falls into a fire or into water. I brought him to your disciples, but none of them could heal him."

Jesus said, "You people are too stubborn to have any faith! How much longer must I be with you? Why do I have to put up with you? Bring the boy here." Then Jesus spoke sternly to the demon. It went out of the boy, and right then he was healed.

Later the disciples went to Jesus in private and asked him, "Why couldn't we force out the demon?"

Jesus replied: "It is because you don't have enough faith! But I can promise you this. If you had faith no larger than a mustard seed, you could tell this mountain to move from here to there. And it would. Everything would be possible for you. [But the only way to force out this kind of demon is by praying and going without eating.]" (Some manuscripts add this last, bracketed statement. See also Mark 9:14-29 and Luke 9:37-42.)

 Focus on the Scripture

The Gospel accounts of Matthew, Mark, and Luke all report that prior to this healing, Jesus and three of his disciples had gone up on a mountain by themselves for a brief retreat. This turned out to be one of the most amazing spiritual highlights of their lives. All four of them heard the voice of God say, "This is my Son, the Beloved; with him I am well pleased; listen to him!" (Matt. 17:5, NRSV). The ecstasy and euphoria of that event soon evaporated when they returned to the crowd below and were confronted with an upset father, his very sick son, and frustrated disciples.

You may question Jesus' habit of going off alone or with his close friends, leaving masses of hurting, helpless, unhealed people. Sometimes people must retreat in order to go forward. As the saying goes, "Come apart or you will fall apart." Jesus obviously needed personal time for spiritual renewal, and so do you. His demonstrated effectiveness in ministering to people is directly linked to his personal prayer life. Likewise, time that you spend alone with God is not wasted and enables you to be more helpful to others later on.

To return to the story, we find the mountaintop high followed by problems in the valley below. The disappointed father appealed directly to Jesus, stating that the disciples had tried but failed to heal his son. Matthew 17:17 clearly indicates that Jesus expected his disciples to be much more effective in his absence. You can sense Jesus' frustration rising almost to the point of exploding at the hapless healers, as he criticizes them for their faithlessness and lack of understanding, even though they have been living with him day after day.

Jesus then healed the boy of his epilepsy, using the therapy of deliverance by commanding the evil spirit to leave. *Epilepsy* comes from the Greek word for "seizure." Medical research today says that an epileptic person has a brain disorder affecting the nervous system, usually characterized by fits of convulsions that end with loss of consciousness. Epilepsy can be hereditary or brought on by trauma. It is treatable but not curable, sometimes going into a state of remission.

When the disciples questioned Jesus as to why they were not successful in helping the boy, Jesus admitted that this kind of illness was difficult to control and to cure. The spiritual therapy advised by Jesus in Matthew 17:20-21 is an unwavering faith, much prayer, and, according to some manuscripts of this text, going without food (fasting). This instructional word from Jesus also applies to present-day Christians who feel called into healing ministry. Nothing more nor less is required than a personal commitment to a life of prayer and sacrificial living, based on the foundation of faith in God's caring compassion as revealed in Jesus.

Some may question the validity and value of fasting from food and drink. How can voluntary abstinence for a temporary period have a noticeable spiritual impact? The Bible contains nearly one hundred references to fasting. Those who have engaged in self-imposed fasts attest to these benefits:

- promotes a positive outlook with a Christlike perspective;

- heightens sensitivity to the needs of others, clarifying motivation to serve;

- directs attention away from personal needs and fosters concentration on God's will and purposes;

- offers a gift of time that would have been spent in meal preparation and eating.

One must experience the spiritual discipline of fasting in order to realize and explain the benefits.

A Reading to Think About

BY HARVEY AND LOIS SEIFERT

An ancient saying suggested that there are two wings by which we rise, one being personal piety and the other community charity. No one can fly by flapping only one wing. It is impossible to be sincere in our worship of God without expecting to do the will of God. It is equally impossible to do the full will of God without the guidance and empowerment of a vital personal relationship with God. As Allan Hunter has said, "Those who picket should also pray, and those who pray should also picket." The same combination of devotional vitality and social action is also emphasized in the two great commandments of Jesus—to love God with all one's being and to love other persons as ourselves (Matt. 22:36-40).[35]

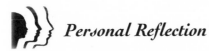 *Personal Reflection*

What is God saying to you in this story?

1. Carefully read and reread the scripture passage. Write down any thoughts, ideas, and questions that may come to you. Do not hurry.

2. Name the specific illness or problem in this story and list all factors that seemed to work together for healing.

117

3. Come apart or you will fall apart. What would it take for you to come away from your everyday, unrelenting stress and worries for periods of personal rest and renewal? Right now block out a brief time period each day, a more extended time once a week, plus a half or full day each month. Opportunities abound for overnight and weekend spiritual retreats. Experience these refreshing times of coming apart until you discover what works best for you. Ask God to help you with this exploration.

4. In this healing story, Jesus was impressed with the won't-take-no-for-an-answer faith of the boy's father. However, Jesus was not impressed with his own faithless disciples. On a scale of 1 to 10, with 10 being 100 percent confident in the active presence of the Healing Christ, what number value would you give your personal faith at this very moment? In Mark's version of this story, the father says to Jesus, "I believe; help my unbelief!" (Mark 9:24, NRSV). What does this verse mean to you?

5. Perhaps you feel powerless to help certain people in your life whom you love and care for deeply. In addition to praying for each one each day, you could engage in the spiritual discipline of fasting for a predetermined length of time. Prayer coupled with fasting could reveal insights and possible help-

ful steps. You may want to experiment with this combination of disciplines repeatedly, recording your thoughts, feelings, and results each time.

Caring Prayer for Others

Lovingly and thankfully lift in prayer those persons in your life who seem to be powerless to enjoy good health, whether physical, mental, or spiritual.

Resting in God's Presence

Now put aside your personal agenda and simply relax, basking in the warmth and healing light of God's love.

Go forth from this special place knowing that the grace and peace of Christ go with you!

19

BLINDNESS: PHYSICAL AND SPIRITUAL

Centering Prayer

O God of light and life, as the psalmist prayed, so I now affirm that "even the darkness is not dark to you; / the night is as bright as the day, / for darkness is as light to you" (Ps. 139:12, NRSV). May the light of Christ illuminate our time together, dispelling any darkness and giving clarity to what you say to me today. Amen.

Holy Scripture

JOHN 9:1-11

As Jesus walked along, he saw a man who had been blind since birth. Jesus' disciples asked, "Teacher, why was this man born blind? Was it because he or his parents sinned?"

"No, it wasn't!" Jesus answered. "But because of his blindness, you will see God work a miracle for him. As long as it is day, we must do what the one who sent me wants me to do. When night comes, no one can work. While I am in the world, I am the light for the world."

After Jesus said this, he spit on the ground. He made some mud and smeared it on the man's eyes. Then he said, "Go and wash off the mud in Siloam Pool." The man went and washed in Siloam, which means "One Who Is Sent." When he had washed off the mud, he could see.

The man's neighbors and the people who had seen him begging wondered if he really could be the same man. Some of them said he was the same beggar, while others said he only looked like him. But he told them, "I am that man."

"Then how can you see?" they asked.

He answered, "Someone named Jesus made some mud and smeared it on my eyes. He told me to go and wash it off in Siloam Pool. When I did, I could see." (Read the entire ninth chapter of John's Gospel for the full context and impact of this healing story.)

 Focus on the Scripture

Recorded only in John's Gospel, this fascinating healing story teaches us that those who do not place their complete faith and trust in Jesus live in spiritual darkness. Those who do believe in Jesus, accepting his teachings as God's truth, have spiritual vision and understanding. In the key verse, "I am the light for the world" (John 9:5), Jesus clearly identifies himself as God's Son sent to illuminate and dispel the darkness. This teaching is reinforced later in the story (John 9:35-41).

Healing the man who was born blind is a dramatic and highly effective way of saying to the skeptical disciples, neighbors, Pharisees, and parents (as well as to all who read this passage) that spiritual blindness is far worse than physical blindness. The author of this Gospel records some popular misconceptions and negative attitudes regarding the connection between sin and sickness.

Jesus' disciples express the problem according to conventional wisdom of that day: "Teacher, why was this man born blind? Was it because he or his parents sinned?" (John 9:2). Certainly we can bring on some illnesses by way of unhealthy habits and personal sin, but Jesus states that is not the case in this man's situation: "Neither this man nor his parents sinned" (John 9:3, NRSV). We like that part of Jesus' answer, but countless readers fasten onto the next part and ignore the main teaching. Jesus replied, "But because of his blindness, you will see God work a miracle for him" (John 9:3).

A seminary professor told his class one day that whenever he came upon a passage in the Bible that made no sense or was beyond his understanding, he would make this note in the margin: "Awaiting further light." It is okay not to have an answer to every question raised in reading the Bible. Human limitations and lack of helpful knowledge often hinder us. Through shared Bible study, personal research, the insights of other persons, and prayers for the enlightenment of the Holy Spirit, additional light often is shed on formerly obscure passages.

What about John 9:3? Does this verse imply that God caused this man to be born blind so that Jesus could perform a teaching miracle at the appropriate moment? Does this statement mean that all birth defects have a purpose known only to God? Does this comment underscore the mystery of human sickness and disabling conditions? Answer: awaiting further light!

Let us focus on the actions and reactions of the man who was given new eyes and the gift of spiritual vision.

- He did not ask Jesus to heal his blindness.

- No one brought him to Jesus for healing.

- Jesus took the initiative and gained the man's confidence by using spittle to make a mud cake for the man's eyes. Saliva was believed to have healing characteristics.

- The man then obediently followed Jesus' instructions by washing himself in the pool of Siloam.

- When the man began telling everyone he could now see, the neighbors did not rejoice but expressed disbelief.

- The neighbors took the man to the Pharisees, who also exhibited skepticism.

- The Pharisees brought in the man's parents to verify the alleged miracle.

- Everyone demanded an explanation, but the sighted man could only say, "All I know is that I used to be blind, but now I can see!" (John 9:25).

An understanding Sunday-school teacher told her class of adults who were asking difficult questions about Jesus: "Always remember that nowhere in the Bible does Jesus say, 'Explain me.' He just says, 'Follow me.'"

A Reading to Think About

BY LARRY DOSSEY, M.D.

Our understanding of the relationship between spirituality and healing is vastly incomplete. We should admit the obvious: *There is great mystery here.* By "mystery" I do not mean temporary ignorance that will later be swept away by additional information, or questions that will someday be resolved by future research. I mean mystery in the strongest possible sense—something unknowable, something essentially beyond human understanding. The fact that saints sometimes suffer and sinners don't is but one expression of this mystery. . . .

Mystery irritates; it demands solutions. Perhaps this is because we are so intolerant of ambiguity, generally preferring things in black or white without shades of gray. When faced with mystery, we often engage in desperate attempts to solve it. . . .

If we are ever to understand the role of prayer in healing, and the relationship between spirituality and health, we shall have to grow more tolerant of ambiguity and mystery. We shall have to be willing to stand in the unknown.[36]

 Personal Reflection

What is God saying to you in this healing story?

1. Carefully read and reread the scripture passage. Write down any thoughts, ideas, and questions that may come to you.

2. Name the specific illness or problem in this story and list all factors that seemed to work together for healing.

3. "Awaiting further light!" What are some biblical questions, issues, events, or passages that leave you in the dark? Name them. Write them down. Discuss them with other Christians. Pray over them and pray for the light of Christ to illuminate your questing spirit and mind as you await further light.

4. What do you make of the parents' reaction to the news that their adult son was no longer blind (see John 9:18-23)? Imagine you are that adult son. Write out your response to your parents that day.

5. The character and nature of God, as revealed by Jesus, inform us that God does not inflict us with life-threatening illnesses, critical accidents, or handicapping disabilities. However, in all situations, conditions, and circumstances, God is able to work for good, bringing blessings, hope, and help. As the apostle Paul wrote, "We know that all things work together for good for those who love God, who are called according to his purpose" (Rom. 8:28, NRSV). Name a recent personal trauma or tragedy that you could offer to God in prayer right now, patiently waiting and fully expecting some good to come out of it all.

Caring Prayer for Others

Lift by name in prayer those you know who have a restless need to explain all the unanswered questions in the Bible and in their personal lives.

Resting in God's Presence

Now put aside your personal agenda and simply relax, basking in the warmth and healing light of God's love.

Go forth from this special place knowing that the grace and peace of Christ go with you!

20

THE SENSITIVITY OF JESUS

Centering Prayer

> O God, you are my God, I seek you,
>> my soul thirsts for you;
> my flesh faints for you,
>> as in a dry and weary land where there is no water.
> So I have looked upon you in the sanctuary,
>> beholding your power and glory.
> Because your steadfast love is better than life,
>> my lips will praise you.
> So I will bless you as long as I live;
>> I will lift up my hands and
>>> call on your name (Ps. 63:1-4, NRSV).

Holy Scripture

MARK 7:31-37

Jesus left the region around Tyre and went by way of Sidon toward Lake Galilee. He went through the land near the ten cities known as Decapolis. Some people brought to him a man who was deaf and could hardly talk. They begged Jesus just to touch him.

After Jesus had taken him aside from the crowd, he stuck his fingers in the man's ears. Then he spit and put it on the man's tongue. Jesus looked up toward heaven, and with a groan he said, "Effatha!" which means "Open up!" At once the man could hear, and he had no more trouble talking clearly.

Jesus told the people not to say anything about what he had done. But the more he told them, the more they talked about it. They were completely amazed and said, "Everything he does is good! He even heals people who cannot hear or talk."

 ## *Focus on the Scripture*

Because Jesus understood the complexities of human nature, he did not offer the same kind of healing help to everyone who came to him. Some he healed through laying on his hands; some were cured without physical touch. With some Jesus prayed silently; with others he offered a spoken word. Some were helped by Jesus' visiting in their homes; others Jesus healed without making a "house call." Sometimes he mentioned the importance of faith; sometimes he did not.

No one can accuse Jesus of being a mechanistic healer, an assembly-line physician with little regard for the dignity, the feelings, and the uniqueness of each person. Here, in this tender, intimate healing story recorded only in Mark's Gospel, we see a picture of Jesus, the kind, courteous, creative Healer. Here was a man with a speech impediment and severe hearing loss. His friends brought him to Jesus with but one request: "They begged Jesus just to touch him" (Mark 7:32).

Notice Jesus' sensitivity at this point. Before proceeding, he took the man aside. The Good News Translation of the Bible reads: "So Jesus took him off alone, away from the crowd" (Mark 7:33). Get the picture? This is a private healing, only two people, Jesus and the man who was deaf and who could hardly talk. Would this privacy have removed some embarrassment? Yes. Would the man have appreciated the sign language Jesus used in the actual healing process? Yes. Would the man have been repulsed when Jesus placed a small amount of his spittle on the man's tongue? No. Popular belief in those days held that saliva contained healing agents. Then, with an authoritative command, Jesus spoke the healing words, "Open up!" At once the man was able to hear and his speech impediment was gone. Praise God!

In reading this story, you get the feeling that Mark left out a line that would explain how Jesus and the cured man moved from "private" back to "public." In Mark 7:36 Jesus cautioned the people not to say anything about what he had done that day. This could mean that the man who no longer had the limitations of deafness and speech disability was so excited and happy that he just had to go back and tell his friends, who in turn told others. If you have ever been healed of a disabling condition or a life-threatening illness, did you not want to tell the whole world? It's hard to contain the good news of restored health and new life!

Perhaps you noticed the similarity of this healing story to the one in Matthew 12:22-28 (see meditation 15, "Protection from Evil"). Two significant differences emerge: (1) the man in the other story was blind and mute; (2) in the other story, the people said the man had a demon in him. Demons and evil spirits are not mentioned in Mark 7:31-37. Nor does the word *sin* appear in this story. We cannot assign cause or blame for every illness to the devil or to personal sin. At times our sinful habits do bring on personal unhealthiness, and evil does have the capability to make us sick. Even though we may not be able to explain the genesis of every sickness, we do know who is more than able to help us deal with our personal unhealthiness: the loving, compassionate, sensitive, creative Healer and Savior, the Lord Jesus Christ!

In several healing stories, Jesus told the people to keep the healing quiet and not to pass on news about it. Why the requested secrecy? One explanation says that Jesus was simply using reverse psychology. If you want people to do something, tell them not to do it. A more acceptable theory holds that Jesus did not want to be known primarily as a fantastic healer. His main mission was to preach and to teach: "'The right time has come,'" he said, "'and the Kingdom of God is near! Turn away from your sins and believe the Good News!'" (Mark 1:15, GNT).

The healing ministry of Jesus is positive evidence that God's reign and realm are real!

A Reading to Think About

BY JIM GLENNON

Christ healed because it was God's will; he healed because of his compassion; he healed to fulfill prophecy; he healed to confirm his Messiahship and his power to forgive sins; he healed to give glory to God; he healed to bring people to believe in him as Lord; and he healed in response to faith. . . .

The reason the Son of God appeared was to destroy the works of the devil.[37]

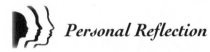 *Personal Reflection*

What is God saying to you in this story?

1. Carefully read and reread the scripture passage. Write down any thoughts, ideas, and questions that may come to you. Do not hurry.

2. Name the specific illness or problem in this story and list all factors that seemed to work together for healing.

3. Jesus consistently offered sensitivity, compassion, and courtesy to persons who were ill, in pain, hurt, or abused. What is your attitude toward those who are less than healthy? How do you act in the presence of sickness?

4. The man in this story was limited by hearing and speaking disabilities. Everyone is limited in one way or another. Make a list of your personal limitations (physical, mental, spiritual, and in relationship with others). Are you living creatively within your limitations? Are you seeking the spiritual therapy of Christ to help you overcome or to cope with your limitations?

5. Make a list of your strengths, abilities, and God-given talents and gifts. Offer a sincere prayer of thanksgiving for who you are as a unique child of God. What are some ways you are using your strengths in serving God?

Caring Prayer for Others

With the respectful sensitivity of Jesus, pray by name for persons you know who are living with embarrassing or socially unacceptable kinds of illnesses.

Resting in God's Presence

Now put aside your personal agenda and simply relax, basking in the warmth and healing light of God's love.

Go forth from this special place knowing that the grace and peace of Christ go with you!

21

SICK WITH A FEVER

Centering Prayer

Your Son, Jesus, amazes me, O God, when I am reminded that no human need, small or great, was beyond his caring compassion. As I meet with you right now, encourage me to bring my personal needs, both small and great, to Jesus, my Savior and Healer. Amen.

Holy Scripture

MATTHEW 8:14-15

Jesus went to the home of Peter, where he found that Peter's mother-in-law was sick in bed with fever. He took her by the hand, and the fever left her. Then she got up and served Jesus a meal. (See also Mark 1:29-31 and Luke 4:38-39.)

 Focus on the Scripture

This touching vignette in Jesus' busy life offers us insight and encouragement. Recorded by Matthew, Mark, and Luke, this brief healing encounter with Peter's mother-in-law speaks volumes. Although Luke's version is slightly different, all three agree

- that Jesus went home one day with Peter,
- that Jesus was directed to Peter's mother-in-law, who was sick in bed with a fever,

❧ that Jesus helped her by getting rid of the fever,

❧ that the woman got up and served Jesus immediately.

While this healing does not appear to be as dramatic as some in the Gospels, nevertheless a fever is not to be taken lightly or to be ignored. The word *fever* is akin to the Latin for *warm*. When you have a fever, you have an abnormal rise in your body temperature. A fever is an easily recognized symptom pointing to a potentially serious condition. A fever gets our attention. A fever can be high or low. Luke says the woman "was sick with a high fever."

This short story does not indicate that the woman asked for Jesus to come heal her. We can well imagine that other family members asked Jesus to see what he could do to help her. We have no dialogue between Jesus and the woman. Even though the faith factor is not mentioned, we can assume that Jesus always had faith in his heavenly Father to intervene in every situation, and we probably could assume that being related to Peter, this woman would have had some degree of expectation that Jesus could help her.

When we read the verses in Matthew 8 leading up to this story, we see that Jesus was in the midst of a hectic agenda that day. He must have been hungry, tired, and exhausted upon entering Peter's house. Yet his ever-present compassion outweighed his personal agenda as he focused on the needs of Peter's mother-in-law.

The mother-in-law reacted to the relief from fever by getting out of bed to serve Jesus food. Wanting to express gratitude for help and healing from Jesus is a typical response, even today. Whenever you feel and truly believe that Jesus has touched your life in a personal and positive manner, you naturally want to serve him.

A Reading to Think About

BY TILDA NORBERG AND ROBERT D. WEBBER

In the New Testament we read many stories of people bringing loved ones to Jesus for healing or coming to Jesus on behalf of others. . . .

While it is very natural to pray earnestly for our loved ones in need, we can learn ways to channel our natural compassion that will make for more effective praying. Here are some ways to help get ourselves out of the way so that the Lord can work in and through us.

It is important to let go of rules and techniques, so God will have room to work. Much of the spiritual preparation for healing prayer has to do with knowing our helplessness and emptiness on the one hand, and God's overflowing love and mercy on the other. Prayer for healing means inviting God to work in the person in God's own way.[38]

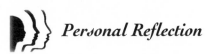 *Personal Reflection*

What is God saying to you in this story?

1. Carefully read and reread the scripture passage. Write down any thoughts, ideas, and questions that may come to you. Do not hurry.

2. Name the specific illness or problem in this story and list all factors that seemed to work together for healing.

3. Have you or a loved one ever been sick with a fever? It can be scary not knowing what's causing this sign of sickness.

133

Name the steps you take to get rid of a fever. Where on your list do you place prayer and petition to the Healing Christ?

4. Nothing that happens to us is ever beyond or outside Christ's personal concern and loving compassion. What are you concerned about, anxious about, worried about today? Name your concerns, and take them to the Lord in prayer.

5. After the woman in this story was healed, she got up and served Jesus. Has your life been touched in any way by the healing grace of Jesus? If so, how are you expressing your gratitude? In what ways are you serving Jesus?

Caring Prayer for Others

Just as family members called Jesus' attention to Peter's mother-in-law, so you have the privilege and opportunity to invite Jesus to give special attention to your family members. Lovingly name them and lift them into the light and love of Jesus.

Resting in God's Presence

Now put aside your personal agenda and simply relax, basking in the warmth and healing light of God's love.

Go forth from this special place knowing that the grace and peace of Christ go with you!

22

GRADUAL IMPROVEMENT

Centering Prayer

Knowing that you are always receptive to the prayer of faith, Lord Jesus, I come to you now in faith and trust, believing that your caring compassion is powerfully present. Amen.

Holy Scripture

JOHN 4:46-53

While Jesus was in Galilee, he returned to the village of Cana, where he had turned the water into wine. There was an official in Capernaum whose son was sick. And when the man heard that Jesus had come from Judea, he went and begged him to keep his son from dying.

Jesus told the official, "You won't have faith unless you see miracles and wonders!"

The man replied, "Lord, please come before my son dies!"

Jesus then said, "Your son will live. Go on home to him." The man believed Jesus and started back home. Some of the official's servants met him along the road and told him, "Your son is better!" He asked them when the boy got better, and they answered, "The fever left him yesterday at one o'clock."

The boy's father realized that at one o'clock the day before, Jesus had told him, "Your son will live!" So the man and everyone in his family put their faith in Jesus.

Focus on the Scripture

This story, found only in John's Gospel, has several features that get our attention. First of all, parents and grandparents immediately feel a bond of empathy with the father. Here is a man of high position in the court system, identified simply as an official or a nobleman He has come from Capernaum to Cana, approximately twenty miles, to get help from Jesus for his dying son. Jesus' first words sound like a disparaging remark to the desperate father: "You won't have faith unless you see miracles and wonders!" Actually the Greek word for *you* in this sentence is plural, meaning Jesus was addressing the father and the onlookers. Jesus already had a miracle worker's reputation in of Cana, where he had previously changed water into wine at a wedding. (See John 2:1-11.)

Obviously the father was not there out of curiosity, and he repeated his plea, "Lord, please come before my son dies!" Notice Jesus did not go home with him. Jesus did not make house calls every time someone came to him for help. He instructed the distraught father to go home because, said Jesus, "Your son will live." The true faith of the father was revealed when he did not ask Jesus a third time to come to his house; rather he believed Jesus and started back home.

Those who pray regularly for the healing love of Jesus to touch people in near and faraway places are not surprised when the father is greeted by his servants with the wonderful news, "Your son is better!" The father discovered that the fever had left the boy at the very same time Jesus said, "Your son will live." The father's faith was affirmed, and all in the family became believers in Jesus.

Another point to underline in this story is the phrase in John 4:52, "the boy got better." Other translations say, "He began to recover" (NRSV); "he began to mend" (RSV). No instant cure in this case but rather a noticeable improvement. Faith and prayer speed up the healing process. At times recovery is instantaneous, but most often healing comes with gradual improvement. Getting sick is a process and getting well again is a process.

A Reading to Think About

BY FRANCIS MACNUTT

Just to know that healing is a mystery—that it's complicated and not all that simple—should free us from any need to give simplistic answers to people who wonder why they are not totally healed. To know how complex healing is helps us to rely more upon God's light, to seek real discernment, and to let go of simplified solutions.[39]

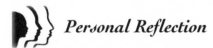 *Personal Reflection*

What is God saying to you in this story?

1. Carefully read and reread the scripture passage. Write down any thoughts, ideas, and questions that may come to you. Do not hurry.

2. Name the specific illness or problem in this story and list all factors that seemed to work together for healing.

3. Notice that the father in this story made an intentional journey to seek spiritual help. His bold initiative in going to Jesus becomes a model for us. When you or a loved one gets sick,

whom do you seek for healing? What priority do you give to the Risen Christ and his desire to help and to heal?

4. What are some ways you can live your faith in Christ every day?

5. Gradual improvement is not as dramatic as total remission or complete healing but still is undeniable evidence that God's healing grace and power are always available to us. List times when you prayed for an immediate cure, only to experience healing at a slower pace. Express prayers of gratitude for God's past, present, and future healing in your life.

Caring Prayer for Others

O Christ, Divine Physician and Savior, make me more sensitive to all who are bound together in the fellowship of suffering. Right now I bring to you by name these persons for your help and healing. [*Pray for each one by name.*] Thank you for helping and healing. Amen.

Resting in God's Presence

Now put aside your personal agenda and simply relax, basking in the warmth and healing light of God's love.

Go forth from this special place knowing that the grace and peace of Christ go with you!

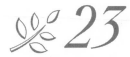

TOUCHED A SECOND TIME

Centering Prayer

Calm me down, O God. Center my spirit in you and help me to be fully present to your loving presence during these precious moments alone with you. Amen.

Holy Scripture

MARK 8:22-26

As Jesus and his disciples were going into Bethsaida, some people brought a blind man to him and begged him to touch the man. Jesus took him by the hand and led him out of the village, where he spit into the man's eyes. He placed his hands on the blind man and asked him if he could see anything. The man looked up and said, "I see people, but they look like trees walking around."

Once again Jesus placed his hands on the man's eyes, and this time the man stared. His eyes were healed, and he saw everything clearly. Jesus said to the man, "You may return home now, but don't go into the village."

 Focus on the Scripture

This story is found only in the Gospel of Mark. Clearly Jesus had great compassion and sensitivity for persons with impaired eyesight. Notice the kindness and caring of Jesus. He respected the blind man's dignity by taking him by the hand and leading him out of the village, away from curious onlookers. Then Jesus used a healing method that seems strange to us but not to the man in the story: "He spit into the man's eyes." "Spittle therapy" helped this man to be more at ease with Jesus, who spoke and acted in ways people could understand.

What makes this story unique is the second touch by Jesus after the first treatment brought only partially restored vision. This is neither an insult to his healing power nor a reflection on the blind man's initial response. Rather here is an undeniable word of encouragement to all of us who do not experience an immediate cure but do notice some improvement in our condition. Is healing in stages any less of a miracle than an instantaneous cure? One may be more dramatic, but God's grace is working in every timetable for healing.

This story encourages us to go to the Healing Christ repeatedly to pray about the same sickness. We would do well to remember the wisdom of the Quaker philosopher Elton Trueblood: "Whatever is worth worrying about is worth praying about."[40]

Probably the blind man would have been pleased to receive partial sight. Do you sometimes settle too quickly for a temporary improvement, or do you creatively explore several options that could be helpful in the healing process? Christ yearns for each of us to be whole and completely healthy, but often we give up too soon or are satisfied with less than complete healing.

A Reading to Think About

BY CATHERINE MARSHALL

Jesus came to earth to reveal His Father's nature and His will for [humankind]. Jesus saw sickness and disease as intruders in His Father's world, part of Satan's work, therefore evil all the way. Consistently Jesus fought disease just as any dedicated physician fights it. . . .

He did not once say in regard to health, "If it is God's will." There is no beatitude for the sick as there is for others like the bereaved, those who suffer persecution, the peacemakers. Nor did there ever fall from Jesus' lips any statements that ill health would further our spiritual growth or benefit the kingdom of God. Rather, He not only wants to heal our diseases, He also wants us to stay healthy.[41]

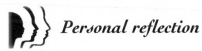 *Personal reflection*

What is God saying to you in this story?

1. Carefully read and reread the scripture passage. Write down any thoughts, ideas, and questions that may come to you. Do not hurry.

2. Name the specific illness or problem in this story and list all factors that seemed to work together for healing.

3. This story teaches us that it is okay to pray more than once about a sickness that does not go away quickly. Name a time or two when you asked for an instant miracle but experienced gradual healing. Reflect on your reactions.

4. Do you sometimes settle too quickly for temporary improvement? Perhaps God is speaking to you and challenging you to become more assertive in exploring other options in the healing process. Record any thoughts, feelings, and promptings of the Holy Spirit.

5. Continue your prayer time with God as you would engage in conversation with your best friend, remembering that you do not need to do all the talking. Allow God's gentle, healing presence to touch you a second time or more.

Caring Prayer for Others

Pray by name for those you know who are dealing with chronic pain and recurring sickness.

Resting in God's Presence

Now put aside your personal agenda and simply relax, basking in the warmth and healing light of God's love.

Go forth from this special place knowing that the grace and peace of Christ go with you!

24

TELL JESUS WHAT YOU WANT

Centering Prayer

O God, even as people in the Gospel stories did not hesitate to call out to your Son, Jesus, to get his attention and to seek his help, so I come to you in this sacred place for our special time together. Give me clarity to see and to know what I need more than anything else right now. I come in humble boldness to ask for your divine assistance and with the genuine desire to follow Jesus with joyful obedience. Amen.

Holy Scripture

MATTHEW 20:29-34

Jesus was followed by a large crowd as he and his disciples were leaving Jericho. Two blind men were sitting beside the road. And when they heard that Jesus was coming their way, they shouted, "Lord and Son of David, have pity on us!"

The crowd told them to be quiet, but they shouted even louder, "Lord and Son of David, have pity on us!"

When Jesus heard them, he stopped and asked, "What do you want me to do for you?" They answered, "Lord, we want to see!"

Jesus felt sorry for them and touched their eyes. Right away they could see, and they became his followers.

Focus on the Scripture

This incident in Jesus' public life demonstrates again his special sensitivity to persons who were visually challenged. Notice that the two blind men took the initiative in getting Jesus' attention by shouting loudly at him. It was the custom in those days for visiting rabbis to teach as they walked along with anyone who cared to listen. Because large numbers constantly crowded around Jesus, he would not have been aware of two unsighted men sitting by the side of the road. Their somewhat drastic and discourteous attempt to get a hearing from Jesus was rebuffed severely by the people around them. They were not about to let two beggars break in on their time with the famous teacher from Nazareth.

The rebuff only caused louder shouts from the blind men. They refused to let anyone keep them from Jesus, in whom they displayed a faith that exceeded many sighted persons' that day. Twice they cried out, "Lord and Son of David, have pity on us!" The phrase "Son of David" implied their belief that Jesus was indeed the long-awaited Messiah, sent by God. "Have pity on us" is also translated "Have mercy on us," which is a nonspecific prayer request. Jesus, however, did hear them trying to get his attention. He stopped and told them to be more specific, "What do you want me to do for you?"

Suppose you did not know the next part of this dramatic story. Suppose you did not know exactly what the two blind men wanted. Yes, they asked for mercy and pity, but in what tangible way? They could have been asking for money or food, as most beggars did in those days. Jesus knew what they needed most and what they wanted most, but he felt it necessary for them to verbalize it themselves. "Lord," they answered, "we want to see!"

This insistence on articulating our prayer requests is similar to Jesus' teachings in the Sermon on the Mount (Matt. 5–7). "Ask, and you will receive. Search, and you will find. Knock, and the door will be opened for you" (Matt. 7:7). Yes, God knows what we need without our asking, but God also knows that without our personal desire, cooperation, and appreciation, God's goodness may fall on hardened hearts and unreceptive minds and spirits. Also sometimes we need a cooling-off period after prayer requests are sent Godward in an emotional outburst. Sometimes our own confusion prevents us from knowing what we need. At that point we can prayerfully request insight from the Holy Spirit that will focus our prayer requests as well as increase the hunger of our heart for God's blessed response. Sometimes we do know exactly what we need but are too proud or too stubborn to ask for God's help. It is okay to pray for whatever we need in our personal life. This is why Jesus taught us in his model prayer to say to God, "Give us this day our daily bread" (Matt. 6:11, NRSV).

Upon hearing the two men specify their deep desire to have their eyes opened, Jesus was moved with compassion. He touched their eyes and restored their vision right away. And they became followers, students, learners, disciples, friends of Jesus, and witnesses for Jesus.

A Reading to Think About

BY STEVE HARPER

Give us this day our daily bread. Our prayer leader spoke to God about the needs of the community, the needs of the day, the needs for sustenance. The list in her prayer petition went beyond food, but the message was clear: we are given the privilege of offering up to God the details of our lives. I remember that she also used this section of the pattern in the Lord's Prayer to thank God that we do not have to get everything said at one time—that we would be back tomorrow, and again, and again, asking God's will to be done in the details of our existence. She reminded us to be thankful that God never grows weary of receiving requests about the particulars of our lives.[42]

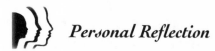 *Personal Reflection*

What is God saying to you in this story?

1. Carefully read and reread the scripture passage. Write down any thoughts, ideas, and questions that may come to you. Do not hurry.

2. Name the specific illness or problem in this story and list all factors that seemed to work together for healing.

3. The crowd tried to keep the blind men from getting Jesus' attention. The crowd stood between Jesus, the Savior and Healer, and the ones who were ready and eager for salvation and healing. What people or obstacles keep you from being with Jesus today?

4. Have you been touched personally by Jesus in your life? Have you known the healing, saving, forgiving presence of God's Son in your personal world? If so, are you actively following Jesus in your life today? Name some ways you express your Christian commitment.

5. The question Jesus asked the two blind men is equally appropriate for everyone who has ever called on him for help in the past or calls on him in the present. Jesus asks, "What do you want me to do for you?" How would you answer Jesus? Before you respond to his question, pray about it, then tell him your answer. Listen prayerfully and carefully for your next step.

Caring Prayer for Others

Close your eyes and ask God to bring names and faces to mind of those whom God wants you to remember at this time. Then thank God for creating and blessing each one. Pray that each one will call upon God for personal needs, situations, and circumstances, knowing that no request is too big or too little to bring to God.

Resting in God's Presence

Now put aside your personal agenda and simply relax, basking in the warmth and healing light of God's love.

Go forth from this special place knowing that the grace and peace of Christ go with you!

25

OPEN MY EYES

Centering Prayer

Open my eyes, that I may see glimpses of truth thou hast for me;
place in my hands the wonderful key that shall unclasp and set
me free.
Silently now I wait for thee, ready, my God, thy will to see.
Open my eyes, illumine me, Spirit divine![43]

Holy Scripture

MARK 10:46-52

Jesus and his disciples went to Jericho. And as they were leaving, they were followed by a large crowd. A blind beggar by the name of Bartimaeus son of Timaeus was sitting beside the road. When he heard that it was Jesus from Nazareth, he shouted, "Jesus, Son of David, have pity on me!" Many people told the man to stop, but he shouted even louder, "Son of David, have pity on me!"

Jesus stopped and said, "Call him over!"

They called out to the blind man and said, "Don't be afraid! Come on! He is calling for you." The man threw off his coat as he jumped up and ran to Jesus.

Jesus asked, "What do you want me to do for you?"

The blind man answered, "Master, I want to see!" Jesus told him, "You may go. Your eyes are healed because of your faith."

Right away the man could see, and he went down the road with Jesus. (See also Luke 18:35-43.)

 Focus on the Scripture

Many New Testament scholars believe this healing story about a blind man named Bartimaeus is basically the same story as recorded in Matthew 20:29-34 (see the previous meditation). Certain similarities are apparent, yet some interesting differences call for our considered attention.

Common to both stories: Jesus and his disciples are leaving Jericho; large crowds follow; a blind man or men shout for Jesus' help; they call Jesus "Son of David," indicating their belief in his messiahship; the crowd tries to quiet the pleas of the blind who cry out a second time; Jesus stops and asks, "What do you want me to do for you?"; the blind respond, "Open our eyes"; Jesus restores their vision, and they become followers.

Now look at the differing details in Mark. Here is a single blind man, identified as Bartimaeus, the son of Timaeus. After he called out loudly to Jesus the second time, Jesus addressed the crowd, "Call him over!" The bystanders stopped harassing and started encouraging the blind man: "Don't be afraid! Come on! He is calling for you." Then the man, elated, jumped up and ran to Jesus, who made a statement not found in the other versions of this story: "Your eyes are healed because of your faith."

In every healing story, faith exists in someone. We can assume that Jesus' activating, circumstance-changing faith in his heavenly Father's love for all humanity permeates every healing scene. The Gospel writers do not consistently describe the faith or faithlessness of others in each case, but one fact is clear: When the person requesting help and healing was a person of faith, Jesus would express his hearty approval with a word of encouragement along with the healing. Our faith in God during times of personal trauma, tragedy, and sickness is therapeutic and gives God more to work with in the healing process.

Bartimaeus is never mentioned again by name in the Bible. The only clue we have about what happened to him is summed up briefly in Mark 10:52: "He went down the road with Jesus."

All three Gospel chroniclers (Matthew, Mark, and Luke) place this story immediately before Jesus' entry into Jerusalem for his triumphal parade and final week of history-changing events. This healing is Jesus' last miracle before his crucifixion and resurrection. Perhaps Bartimaeus had his eyes opened to more than he was prepared to see. What do you think happened to Bartimaeus?

A Reading to Think About

BY ALBERT SCHWEITZER

He [Jesus] comes to us as One unknown, without a name, as of old, by the lake side, He came to those men who knew Him not. He speaks to us the same word: "Follow thou me!" and sets us to the tasks which He has to fulfill for our time. He commands. And to those who obey Him, whether they be wise or simple, He will reveal Himself in the toils, the conflicts, the sufferings which they shall pass through in His fellowship, and, as an ineffable mystery, they shall learn in their own experience Who He is.[44]

 ## Personal Reflection

What is God saying to you in this story?

1. Carefully read and reread the scripture passage. Write down any thoughts, ideas, and questions that may come to you. Do not hurry.

2. Name the specific illness or problem in this story and list all factors that seemed to work together for healing.

3. Reflect on these lines from familiar hymns. How do your personal spiritual experiences compare to those expressed?

   "Open my eyes, that I may see glimpses of truth thou hast for me." (Clara Scott)

   "At the cross, at the cross, where I first saw the light; . . . it was there by faith I received my sight." (Isaac Watts)

   "Amazing grace! How sweet the sound! . . . I once was lost, but now am found; was blind, but now I see." (John Newton)[45]

4. To follow Jesus faithfully means, among other things, to see events, circumstances, and other people with new eyes.

Christians are called to view the world from a Christ-centered perspective. Ask God's Holy Spirit right now to reveal any blind spots in your spiritual vision and understanding.

5. Jesus commended Bartimaeus on his faith. What would Jesus say to you about your faith? Do you live each day by faith or by sight? How does your faith measure up to this description in Hebrews 11:1 (NRSV): "Now faith is the assurance of things hoped for, the conviction of things not seen"? Faith is a gift of the Holy Spirit. If you feel a need to have more confidence in your faith and a boldness to act on your faith, pray expectantly for this to happen.

Caring Prayer for Others

Without being judgmental or critical of others, pray for those you know who seem to suffer from spiritual blindness. Remember, our role is to love others; God's role is to change others. Try not to confuse the two roles.

Resting in God's Presence

Now put aside your personal agenda and simply relax, basking in the warmth and healing light of God's love.

Go forth from this special place knowing that the grace and peace of Christ go with you!

26

THE DEAD ARE RAISED

Centering Prayer

O God, Creator of life here and in the hereafter, help me to have a healthy perspective and understanding in this matter of death. Though I grieve at the graveside of my loved ones, I know that neither life nor death nor anything else in all creation will be able to separate us from your love for everyone in Christ Jesus our Lord. Amen.

Holy Scripture

LUKE 7:11-17

Soon Jesus and his disciples were on their way to the town of Nain, and a big crowd was going along with them. As they came near the gate of the town, they saw people carrying out the body of a widow's only son. Many people from the town were walking along with her. When the Lord saw the woman, he felt sorry for her and said, "Don't cry!"

Jesus went over and touched the stretcher on which the people were carrying the dead boy. They stopped, and Jesus said, "Young man, get up!" The man sat up and began to speak. Jesus then gave him back to his mother.

Everyone was frightened and praised God. They said, "A great prophet is here with us! God has come to his people."

News about Jesus spread all over Judea and everywhere else in that part of the country.

JOHN 11:1-4, 17-19, 33-36, 41-44

A man by the name of Lazarus was sick in the village of Bethany. He had two sisters, Mary and Martha. This was the same Mary who later poured perfume on the Lord's head and wiped his feet with her hair. The sisters sent a message to the Lord and told him that his good friend Lazarus was sick.

When Jesus heard this, he said, "His sickness won't end in death. It will bring glory to God and his Son." . . .

When Jesus got to Bethany, he found that Lazarus had already been in the tomb four days. Bethany was only about two miles from Jerusalem, and many people had come from the city to comfort Martha and Mary because their brother had died. . . .

When Jesus saw that Mary and the people with her were crying, he was terribly upset and asked, "Where have you put his body?"

They replied, "Lord, come and you will see."

Jesus started crying, and the people said, "See how much he loved Lazarus." . . .

After the stone had been rolled aside, Jesus looked up toward heaven and prayed, "Father, I thank you for answering my prayer. I know that you always answer my prayers. But I said this, so that the people here would believe that you sent me." When Jesus had finished praying, he shouted, "Lazarus, come out!" The man who had been dead came out. His hands and feet were wrapped with strips of burial cloth, and a cloth covered his face.

Jesus then told the people, "Untie him and let him go."

 Focus on the Scripture

These two stories raise many questions:

- 🌿 What was the purpose of bringing back to life the widow's son and Lazarus, the brother of Mary and Martha?

- 🌿 Why are these stories in the Bible, and what did the authors intend for readers to learn?

❧ Do these miraculous, pre-Easter healings relate in any way to the ultimate healing in the resurrection of Christ?

❧ When a loved one is pronounced dead, would it be appropriate to pray for that person to be brought back to life?

First of all, we have no biblical records indicating that Lazarus and the widow's son did not die later on in their lives. We must assume that theirs was a temporary reprieve from the undeniable fact that the human race has a 100 percent mortality rate. A clue as to why authors felt it important to include these miracle stories is found in Luke 7:18-23 and Matthew 11:2-6. In these two similar passages, John the Baptizer is in prison and sends two of his disciples to ask Jesus if he indeed is God's Messiah. Jesus replies, "Go and tell John what you have seen and heard: the blind receive their sight, the lame walk, the lepers are cleansed, the deaf hear, the dead are raised, the poor have good news brought to them. And blessed is anyone who takes no offense at me" (Luke 7:22-23, NRSV).

Bringing the dead back to life constitutes indisputable evidence that Jesus is the Christ. John's Gospel reports the raising of Lazarus as one of several signs that enable all to believe in Jesus. However, another significant reason explains inclusion of these stories.

Reread the accounts and notice what they tell us about Jesus the man. In Luke's account, when Jesus and his disciples met the funeral procession that day in the village of Nain, he was informed that the deceased was the only son of his widowed mother. When Jesus saw her, he had compassion for her and said to her, "Do not weep" (Luke 7:13, NRSV). In John's story when Jesus reached the tomb of his good friend Lazarus, Jesus started crying, and the people said, "See how much he loved Lazarus" (John 11:35-36).

The next time you find yourself at the grave of a dear loved one, remember that Jesus, the Christ, knows what you are feeling and experiencing. Our compassionate Savior stands by you and grieves with you, bringing comfort and peace.

Jesus was fully human and fully divine according to the creeds of Christianity, and these two stories well illustrate that truth. In bringing these men back to full life and health, Jesus demonstrates his awesome power and complete authority over death to the amazement of all the bystanders. Those people praised God and said, "A great prophet is here with us! God has come to his people" (Luke 7:16).

Another reason for the inclusion of these stories, as well as the account of Jesus' bringing the twelve-year-old-daughter of Jairus back to life in Luke 8:40-56 (see meditation 12), is to offer a preview of the permanent resurrection of the dead based on the great Easter event. The resurrection of Christ on Easter is a preview of God's intention for everyone, not a short-term resuscitation from the dead but rather ongoing abundant, fully healthy and whole, perfect, eternal life in Christ and with Christ in the heavenly places not prepared by human hands.

Is it appropriate today to pray that God restore life miraculously to those who no longer respond to medical means and heroic efforts of doctors? With the exception of a few successes, many people have made such an attempt only to be devastatingly disappointed. Holy Scripture counsels us to accept our human mortality in this life, as we anticipate what God has prepared for us in the next life. Jesus said to Martha before he brought Lazarus back to life: "I am the resurrection and the life. Those who believe in me, even though they die, will live, and everyone who lives and believes in me will never die" (John 11:25-26, NRSV).

A Reading to Think About

BY RUEBEN P. JOB AND NORMAN SHAWCHUCK

Jesus, who called Lazarus from his tomb and presented him alive to his friends, call me, I pray, from the tombs which seek to stifle the life I have. Remove from me the grave clothes which yet hinder my free movement in your Spirit. Through the power of your name, Amen.[46]

Personal Reflection

What is God saying to you in these stories?

1. Carefully read and reread the scripture passages. Write down any thoughts, ideas, and questions that may come to you. Do not hurry.

2. In these two open-ended stories we are not told what happened to the widow's son or to Lazarus after each regained the breath of life. Let your imagination help you write endings to these two amazing events.

3. "Jesus wept" (John 11:35, KJV). This verse, as it appears in the King James Version, is often noted as the shortest in the Bible. What do these words tell you about Jesus?

4. In what ways have you accepted your own mortality? In what ways could you be in denial about your temporary life on earth?

5. List some of your personal questions and anxieties about death and dying. Then take your thoughts and feelings to God in prayer and listen quietly, remembering that the Risen Christ of Easter has conquered the last enemy, death.

Caring Prayer for Others

Christians grieve just like everyone else over the death of loved ones; however, we do not grieve as those who have no hope. Lift in prayer by name persons you know who are dealing with adjustments and change related to death in their families.

Resting in God's Presence

Now put aside your personal agenda and simply relax, basking in the warmth and healing light of God's love.

Go forth from this special place knowing that the grace and peace of Christ go with you!

27

THE ULTIMATE HEALING

Centering Prayer

In him, who rose from the dead,
our hope of resurrection dawned.
The sadness of death gives way
to the bright promise of immortality.
Lord, for your faithful people life is changed, not ended.[47]
  Amen.

Holy Scripture

JOHN 11:20-27

When Martha heard that Jesus had arrived, she went out to meet him, but Mary stayed in the house. Martha said to Jesus, "Lord, if you had been here, my brother would not have died. Yet even now I know that God will do anything you ask."

Jesus told her, "Your brother will live again!"

Martha answered, "I know that he will be raised to life on the last day, when all the dead are raised." Jesus then said, "I am the one who raises the dead to life! Everyone who has faith in me will live, even if they die. And everyone who lives because of faith in me will never die. Do you believe this?"

"Yes, Lord!" she replied. "I believe that you are Christ, the Son of God. You are the one we hoped would come into the world."

Focus on the Scripture

This is a truly remarkable conversation between Jesus and Martha with its focus on the death of Lazarus, brother to Martha and Mary and a good friend of Jesus. We must marvel at the spiritual insights of Martha, as well as the hope-filled, reassuring words of Jesus spoken today at nearly every funeral and memorial service of a Christian. Said Jesus to Martha—and to everyone who claims him as Lord and Savior—"I am the resurrection and the life. Those who believe in me, even though they die, will live, and everyone who lives and believes in me will never die" (John 11:25-26, NRSV). Keep in mind that this bold affirmation of comfort and hope was spoken before, not after, Easter. The great Easter event of Jesus' resurrection from the grave and return to life actually became the evidence confirming the truth of Jesus' amazing faith-statement to Martha that day.

Health is sometimes discussed in terms of five categories: spiritual, physical, mental, social relationships, and life after death. The first four are temporary, while the fifth and final healing is permanent. Christians understand death of the body as a process one goes through in order to experience the ultimate healing and wholeness in the resurrection of Jesus Christ. Death does not heal; rather, death enables us to make the transition to more life, perfect health, and complete harmony with God.

As I wrote in my earlier book *Blessed to Be a Blessing:*

> Although death, in the minds of many people, is the ultimate tragedy, Christians are heirs of the resurrection of Jesus Christ. This is not to make excuses for what we often perceive as failure in healing before death, or to make slight the deep pain in grieving over the loss of a loved one. This is not to be insensitive to natural fear and ambivalent feelings about the moment of death or the process of dying. Rather, this is an affirmation that only through death and dying can we realize the complete wholeness for which we were created. A person who has had to struggle through life with crippling arthritis, loss of

vision, the burden of brain damage, amputation, or other handicaps may only be fully healed through that transition from life on earth to life in a different state of existence.[48]

Because we highly prize physical fitness and youthful appearances, we expend tremendous amounts of energy, research, and money to improve our physical health. Let us not forget that physically speaking, all human beings are terminal and that all physical healings are temporary. Our Creator God never intended for the human body to function forever. For that reason, we need the broader perspective and appreciation of God's provisions for life after death. These wonderful words of Tommy Tyson's bear repeating now and in times of grief:

> The basis of healing [is] the Incarnation, Crucifixion, and Resurrection. Otherwise, healing is simply a temporary alleviation of a symptom. That's all. But in the light of the resurrection and ascension, healing is a sneak preview of the ultimate. We're going to be changing to His likeness, have a body like unto His own glorious body. Our eyes won't need glasses; our knees won't have arthritis; our tongues won't gossip. We are going to have a resurrected body like unto His own. That's the glorious foundation for the healing ministry for the Church.[49]

A Reading to Think About

BY ANNE S. WHITE

Jesus revealed in His own death and resurrection the Good News that death is only the means of entering into a larger and more wonderful life planned for us; "whoever believes in me shall never die." Eternal life is ours for the accepting: we become alive in His nearer Presence after we cease to live in this earthly body. We shall see our loved ones again: we shall know and be known. The joy that is set before us will be greater than any known here.

Into Your hands, Lord Jesus, I commend my spirit in perfect trust. Your Peace is now filling me with calm. Amen.[50]

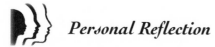 *Personal Reflection*

What is God saying to you in this healing story?

1. Read and reread the scripture passage. Write down any thoughts, ideas, and questions, that may come to you. Do not hurry.

2. Physical death is not the end but the transition to a new chapter in the life of every Christian. Ponder that statement. Record your thoughts.

3. Human nature tends to resist discussions about death and dying. Nevertheless, this would be an appropriate moment to make a list of your fears, anxieties, and unanswered questions surrounding closure to this life and a new life in the hereafter. You may want to make an appointment with a Christian minister to discuss your list.

4. Affirmations and promises regarding our home not made with human hands abound in the Holy Bible. Reflect on this scripture from Revelation 21:1-7, NRSV. Then give thanks to God!

Then I saw a new heaven and a new earth; for the first heaven and the first earth had passed away, and the sea was no more. And I saw the holy city, the new Jerusalem, coming down out of heaven from God, prepared as a bride adorned for her husband. And I heard a loud voice from the throne saying,

"See, the home of God is among mortals.

He will dwell with them as their God;

they will be his peoples,

and God himself will be with them;

he will wipe every tear from their eyes.

Death will be no more;

mourning and crying and pain will be no more,

for the first things have passed away."

And the one who was seated on the throne said, "See, I am making all things new." Also he said, "Write this, for these words are trustworthy and true." Then he said to me, "It is done! I am the Alpha and the Omega, the beginning and the end. To the thirsty I will give water as a gift from the spring of the water of life. Those who conquer will inherit these things, and I will be their God and they will be my children."

5. Revisit the conversation between Jesus and Martha, specifically where Jesus challenges Martha with a penetrating question related to his statement that he is the resurrection and the life and that everyone who believes in him will not die: "[Martha,] do you believe this?" If Jesus were to ask you that question, what would you say? Reread John 11: 25-26. Record your thoughts.

Caring Prayer for Others

Gracious God,
as your son wept with Mary and Martha at the tomb of Lazarus,
look with compassion on those who grieve, [especially *Name(s)*].
Grant them the assurance of your presence now
    and faith in your eternal goodness,
that in them may be fulfilled the promise
    that those who mourn shall be comforted;
through Jesus Christ our Lord. Amen.[51]

Resting in God's Presence

Now put aside your personal agenda and simply relax, basking in the warmth and healing light of God's love.

Go forth from this special place knowing that the grace and peace of Christ go with you!

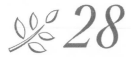 *28*

LARGE CROWDS FOLLOWED JESUS

Centering Prayer

Understanding God, sometimes I feel guilty for repeatedly coming to you for help, yet I know that your Son, Jesus, never turned anyone away. No human need was too small or too big; no problem deemed insolvable; no sickness called incurable. So here I am, once more, grateful for your loving attention. Amen.

Holy Scripture

MARK 6:53-56

Jesus and his disciples crossed the lake and brought the boat to shore near the town of Gennesaret. As soon as they got out of the boat, the people recognized Jesus. So they ran all over that part of the country to bring their sick people to him on mats. They brought them to him each time they heard where he was. In every village or farm or marketplace where Jesus went, the people brought their sick to him. They begged him to let them just touch his clothes, and everyone who did was healed.

MATTHEW 15:29-31

From there, Jesus went along Lake Galilee. Then he climbed a hill and sat down. Large crowds came and brought many people who were crippled or blind or lame or unable to talk. They placed them, and many others, in front of Jesus, and he healed them all. Everyone was amazed at what they saw and heard. People who had never spoken could now speak. The lame were healed, the crippled could walk, and the blind were able to see. Everyone was praising the God of Israel. (See also Luke 9:10-11; Matt. 14:13-14, 34-36; 19:1-2.)

 ## *Focus on the Scripture*

Human nature has not changed in the many hundreds of years since Jesus walked this earth. Today people with so-called incurable illnesses spend extravagant amounts of money to buy newly discovered wonder drugs, travel thousands of miles to check in at world-famous medical clinics, or flock to self-proclaimed faith healers. Personal health problems, disabilities, pain, and suffering rank high on our list of what's most likely to get our undivided attention.

In first-century Israel, desperate people with severe health problems were attracted to Jesus for the same reason. Everywhere he would go, his reputation as an effective, compassionate, amazing healer went ahead of him. The Gospel writers frequently record that large crowds followed Jesus, not primarily for his teaching and preaching but for his ability to cure every disease and infirmity. "When he saw the crowds, [Jesus] had compassion for them, because they were harassed and helpless, like sheep without a shepherd" (Matt. 9:36, NRSV).

The threefold ministry of Jesus is accurately described in the Gospels as preaching, teaching, and healing (see Matt. 4:23 and 9:35). Yet, then as now, his followers tend to emphasize one ministry to the exclusion of the other two. Some people today see Jesus primarily as a great preacher, a God-sent Savior who died on the cross for the sins of the world and who has saved believers from death to eternal life. Some see Jesus primarily as a master teacher, whose recorded words contain all the wisdom and guidance necessary for a satisfying, productive, fulfilled life. Some see Jesus primarily as a healer, a spiritual doctor whose curing power, love, and compassion do not fail in times of personal distress, disease, and disappointment. I once heard a wise woman in the church put all of this in an easy-to-remember perspective:

"Preaching proclaims the gospel. Teaching explains the gospel. Healing makes real the gospel."

Jesus was so popular with the masses that he easily could have used his healing powers as a stepping-stone to personal ambitions. Indeed this very temptation was faced and overcome by Jesus early in his ministry (see Matt. 4:1-11). Even though Jesus' genuine sensitivity to human need caused him to feed large groups of hungry people and to engage in compassionate healing everywhere he went, he never lost focus on his number one mission as recorded in Mark 1:14-15: "Jesus came to Galilee, proclaiming the good news of God, and saying, 'The time is fulfilled, and the kingdom of God has come near; repent, and believe in the good news'" (NRSV).

Throughout his life Jesus held fast to his allegiance to God, empowering people to be reconciled, forgiven, joyful children of God. In his preaching, teaching, and healing, Jesus modeled a balanced, holistic way of life. Jesus never turned away anyone who came for healing. Likewise, you need never hesitate to go to him when you or your loved ones are dealing with sickness. Jesus wants you to bring to him more than your problems and illnesses, however. He also asks—insists—that his followers give him absolute obedience, 100 percent loyalty, and unwavering commitment every day. Consider this challenging statement from *The United Methodist Book of Worship*:

> God does not promise that we shall be spared suffering but does promise to be with us in our suffering. Trusting that promise, we are enabled to recognize God's sustaining presence in pain, sickness, injury, and estrangement.
>
> Likewise, God does not promise that we will be cured of all illnesses; and we all must face the inevitability of death. . . . The greatest healing of all is the reunion or reconciliation of a human being with God. When this happens, physical healing sometimes occurs, mental and emotional balance is often restored, spiritual health is enhanced, and relationships are healed. For the Christian the basic purpose of spiritual healing is to renew and to strengthen one's relationship with the living Christ.[52]

A Reading to Think About

BY ELTON TRUEBLOOD

The reputation of Christ as a healer had spread so thoroughly that the first word of His arrival caused people to bring the sick to Him on litters. Again the numbers were great and the consequent drain on Christ's powers of compassion was correspondingly great. Important as the act of healing was, we must see it as a diversion from the main task, and almost as a temptation. Christ could have concentrated on healing all of the rest of the available time, and thus avoided the worst enmity of the established leaders, but this activity, valuable as it was to distraught individuals, would have had no enduring effect. The only hope of an enduring effect lay in greater and greater concentration on the redemptive group on the one hand, with eventual challenge of the establishment on the other, in the hope that the miraculous influence of the former would outlive the tragedy of the latter. It may be noted that not one of the mighty acts recorded . . . [in the Gospels] was done with the intention of providing a spectacle at which [people] would wonder. Each act, relating either to nature or to human nature, was done for a reason. The miracles, far from being breaks with world order, were demonstrations of the basic order, the order of God's loving will.[53]

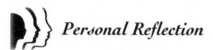 *Personal Reflection*

What is God saying to you in this story?

1. Read and reread the scripture passages. Write down any thoughts, ideas, and questions that may come to you. Do not hurry.

2. Large crowds consistently and constantly followed Jesus. Obviously people came to him for various reasons, many simply out of curiosity. Others wanted only a quick fix for their brokenness or unhealthiness. Some came out of desperation because no one else had been able to help them. Some were not sure why they were drawn to Jesus. Answer these questions: Why am I attracted to Jesus? Why do I call on him? What do I need or want from him? Do I come to Jesus only as the last resort? Perhaps I think of him as a kind of spiritual bellhop always available to respond to my demands.

3. Consider some ways you could apply this biblical truth to your own life: Because Jesus loved the whole person, his goal was to help each person become whole and healthy!

4. When you seek divine healing in your life, do you submit and surrender your total self and your entire personal situation in complete trust and confidence that God loves you dearly and wants only the best for you? When you pray for personal healing, do you share your personal love for God, confessing your sins and knowing God's forgiving grace is

part of the healing process? When you come to God for any reason, do you spend some moments in genuine, personal thanksgiving for all God's blessings in your life? You might want to try these prayer suggestions right now.

5. Jesus came preaching, teaching, and healing. With which of the three types of ministry are you most comfortable? least comfortable? Explore your thoughts and feelings in writing.

Caring Prayer for Others

In prayer you may bring to Jesus friends, family members, and strangers who need his special healing touch. Meditate on the following verse, then pray as the Spirit of Jesus leads you. "Large crowds came and brought many people who were crippled or blind or lame or unable to talk. They placed them, and many others, in front of Jesus, and he healed them all" (Matt. 15:30). Now place before Jesus the names of those you know are in need.

Resting in God's Presence

Now put aside your personal agenda and simply relax, basking in the warmth and healing light of God's love.

Go forth from this special place knowing that the grace and peace of Christ go with you!

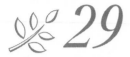

HEALING IN THE NAME OF JESUS

Centering Prayer

Healing Savior, Son of God, cherishing these special moments with you, I center my thoughts and my being on you and in your holy name, Jesus, my Lord. Amen.

Holy Scripture

LUKE 10:1-2, 8-9, 17

Later the Lord chose seventy-two other followers and sent them out two by two to every town and village where he was about to go. He said to them: "A large crop is in the fields, but there are only a few workers. Ask the Lord in charge of the harvest to send out workers to bring it in. . . .

"Heal their sick and say, 'God's kingdom will soon be here!'". . .

When the seventy-two followers returned, they were excited and said, "Lord, even the demons obeyed when we spoke in your name!" (See also Matt. 10:5-15 and Mark 6:7-13.)

 Focus on the Scripture

How did the healing ministry of Jesus get passed on to the ever expanding numbers of Jesus' disciples? How valid is the healing ministry of Jesus for the followers of Jesus today? This significant passage in the Gospel of Luke gives us reliable clues. Early in his public ministry, months before he died, rose from the grave, and ascended into heaven, Jesus began to lay the foundation for his followers to continue all his ministries: teaching, preaching, and healing. Matthew and Mark inform us that Jesus first authorized his twelve apostles to go forth ministering on his behalf. Luke refers to a broader leadership base when he records: "The Lord chose seventy-two other followers and sent them out two by two to every town and village where he was about to go."

Put yourself in the sandals of one of those seventy-two. If you had been one of them, would you have been hesitant, insecure, not overly confident? Probably! But you also would have been more than mildly excited and amazed when you returned from that mission to give a report to your leader. To your great surprise, people responded favorably to your message; the sick got healed; and demons were expelled. How? In the name of Jesus!

Think about that fact. Jesus did not have to be physically present for his ministries to be powerfully effective. The name of Jesus coupled with the sincere, authentic, compassionate availability of his followers made life-changing, positive differences in people's lives. Today's healing ministry works the same way. The basic qualifications for any effective Christian ministry are (1) obedience to Jesus Christ, who instructed his followers to continue all his ministries (see Matt. 28:18-20 and John 14:12-15); (2) compassion and love for other people (see Matt. 22:39 and John 15:12). Francis MacNutt expressed this powerfully simple phenomenon: "You don't have to have any special gift. Just love Jesus and pray for persons—and healing happens. . . . That way seems to work as well as the fantastic gifts of famous faith healers."[54]

A Reading to Think About

BY DONALD BARTOW

The charismatic gift of healing is not a requirement for the Ministry of Healing, but faithfulness on the part of each Christian is the indispensable factor. No special gift of healing is needed for one to begin the Spiritual Healing Ministry because our aim is to lead all to the Great Physician, Jesus Christ. It is not our ability but our availability that is desired. Jesus Christ will do the work and supply the power.[55]

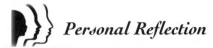 *Personal Reflection*

What is God saying to you in this story?

1. Carefully read and reread the scripture passage. Write down any thoughts, ideas, and questions that may come to you. Do not hurry.

2. Focus on Luke 10:9, which implies a clear connection between personal health and the kingdom of God. As translated in the NRSV, Jesus said, "Cure the sick who are there, and say to them, 'The kingdom of God has come near to you.'" Recall some anxious moments in your past when you or a loved one was cured of a serious illness. You may want to write down these memorable times. Your healing actually was a special sign, factual evidence, that you had experienced the reality of God's kingdom in your life. Pause now to give God the glory. Thank God for those sneak previews of God's kingdom that is already coming on earth as it is in heaven.

3. Notice how Jesus responds to the disciples' victorious report in Luke 10:17-20. He cautions them about the subtle sin of spiritual pride. Can you relate to that warning in your life?

4. If you have been blessed, helped, or healed by praying in the name of Jesus, consider telling others about your personal experiences. Are you in a share-and-prayer group? If not, you could invite two or three of your friends to start one. What are other ways you could more available in leading people to the Great Physician, Jesus Christ?

5. What is God saying to you right now? Is there a special word for you in Luke 10:1-20? If so, write it out.

Caring Prayer for Others

In the precious and powerful name of Jesus, I pray specifically and sincerely for these daughters and sons of God, whom I name right now: [*Names*]. Thank you, Jesus, for giving each one your hope and help and healing. Amen.

Resting in God's Presence

Now put aside your personal agenda and simply relax, basking in the warmth and healing light of God's love.

Go forth from this special place knowing that the grace and peace of Christ go with you!

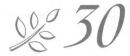 **30**

CHRIST'S HEALING TODAY

Centering Prayer

O God, my Creator, Redeemer, and Sustainer, grant me the peace of Christ in my heart, the wisdom of Christ in my work, the love of Christ in my life, so that I may be a blessing to others and bring glory and honor to you. Amen.

Holy Scripture

JOHN 14:12-14

[Jesus said to his disciples at the Last Supper:] "I tell you for certain that if you have faith in me, you will do the same things that I am doing. You will do even greater things, now that I am going back to the Father. Ask me, and I will do whatever you ask. This way the Son will bring honor to the Father. I will do whatever you ask me to do."

MATTHEW 28:18-20

[After Easter and before ascending into heaven] Jesus came to them and said: "I have been given all authority in heaven and on earth! Go to the people of all nations and make them my disciples. Baptize them in the name of the Father, the Son, and the Holy Spirit, and teach them to do everything I have told you. I will be with you always, even until the end of the world."

HEBREWS 13:8

Jesus Christ never changes! He is the same yesterday, today, and forever.

Focus on the Scripture

One of the most mind-stretching passages in the New Testament is John 14:12-14. Jesus informs his disciples that after he leaves them, they will carry on all his ministries *and* that he expects them to do even greater things for the glory of their heavenly Father. Then forty days after Easter, Jesus gathered them once more before his ascension into heaven. His final words of instruction: "Go to the people of all nations and make them my disciples. Baptize them . . . and teach them to do everything I have told you" (Matt. 28:18-20). We do not lack scriptural authority for Jesus' passing on the ministries of preaching, teaching, and healing to his disciples past, present, and future.

Jesus' commands for continued ministry were never intended only for the original twelve apostles but included everyone who believed in Jesus, had faith in Jesus, and committed their lives in service to Jesus. The number of dedicated followers quickly expanded to 120 (Acts 1:15), to over 3,000 on the day of Pentecost (Acts 2:41), to countless numbers in every nation on the globe today. The best part is that Christians are not spiritual orphans in carrying out our leader's ministries. He is risen! He is with us! He is in the midst of every church community, in every Christian ministry, and in every act of kindness offered in his name. What can we do to be sure we remember those encouraging words of the last sentence in Matthew's Gospel? Said the Risen Christ, "I will be with you always, even until the end of the world" (28:20).

Preaching and teaching ministries rarely have been neglected in the history of Christianity. The healing ministry of the Risen Christ is being rediscovered by twenty-first–century Christians. We are learning to take seriously the authority and presence of Christ in this matter and mystery of healing the whole person: body, mind, spirit, and in human relationships.

The most common expression of Christ's healing ministry today is prayer ministry. When we care about another person, we want to pray for him or her, knowing that our compassion and faith coupled with the compassion and faith of Christ will bless and help. We call upon the presence of the Risen Christ to do the healing. We are not the healers. Likewise, when we come to God in our private times of personal prayer, we have a wonderful opportunity not only to pray for others but to pray for our personal needs as well. Healing ministry is prayer ministry. Prayer ministry is healing ministry.

Everyone prays, but not everyone prays believing that prayer will make a positive difference. The validity of healing prayer is best understood not by rational and intellectual research, as helpful as that can be, but simply by praying. In their book *Stretch Out Your Hand,* Tilda Norberg and Robert Webber state the following:

> *The practice of healing prayer will always be something experienced before it is understood, known by the heart before it is grasped by the mind.* A scientific outlook, legitimate and appropriate in itself, need not be a block to exploring healing prayer. What are needed are a willingness to experiment, an open mind and heart, and trust in God, our good creator and healer.[56]

Jesus' healing ministry, as recorded so faithfully by Matthew, Mark, Luke, and John, reveals that God desires good health for all people. When we pray for healing, for ourselves or for others, we become more receptive and willing to receive what God already has prepared for us in Christ and through the Holy Spirit. Although we do not know *how* prayer works, we do know prayer works. Consider this description of the prayer process:

> Think of prayer as cooperation with God. Think of prayer as giving God permission to move and to act in our lives.
>
> God respects our human freedom. God gave all of us free will to make our own choices in life. In this sense, God patiently waits to offer assistance. Through intentional times of prayer, we give God those grace-filled opportunities.
>
> When we pray for our own healing or the healing of another, we are not in a begging posture; rather, we are intentionally cooperating with God's good will for health, wholeness, and salvation.[57]

A Reading to Think About

BY ALBERT E. DAY

Blessings on you who are seeking to follow in the footsteps of Jesus and to fulfill his command to heal the sick in his name and through his name and through his power. Keep humble. Hold sacred the confidences entrusted to your keeping. Be patient with those who need to come again and again. Guard against the intrusions of well-meaning people who have an unenlightened zeal for God and whose too readily volunteered testimony and exhortation are the source of endless confusion. Let no current skepticisms daunt you. Not everyone will experience the specific healing he or she is seeking, but many will. However, each one will be blessed and helped in some way. Be alert to discover in the unhealed or in their environment or in yourself any hindrances to the renewal of life and seek to clear them away.

This ministry requires constant self-examination and ever larger dedication. Whatever else you do, keep on loving those who need you, those who oppose you, those who fail you. If necessary, lose your life for their sakes and for Christ. So doing you will find life for yourself and for your people on deeper levels. You are Christ's missioner and he will never fail you or your people![58]

 Personal Reflection

What is God saying to you in these stories?

1. Carefully read and reread the scripture passages. Write down any thoughts, ideas, and questions that may come to you. Do not hurry.

2. Through the sacrament of holy baptism Christians are commissioned and empowered for ministry and service in the name of Christ. From the scripture passages in this meditation, we see that Christ fully expects his followers to continue everything he started. Name your special strengths, talents, and gifts. In what ways could you offer your resources to be used in Christ's ministries and for the glory of God? Name any ministry in which you are active. Name some ministries you are not engaged in but have a personal interest in. Perhaps you need to share these thoughts with your pastor. Pray about these matters.

3. Healing ministry is prayer ministry. Prayer ministry is healing ministry. Are you being led into a more intentional prayer and healing ministry, either in your time alone with God or with a small group of other Christians? If so, what might be your next step? Be open to the guidance of the Holy Spirit as you pray about this question.

4. Increasing numbers of pastors and lay leaders in churches today are offering prayer and healing worship services based on the instruction in the Letter of James:

> Are any among you sick? They should call for the elders of the church and have them pray over them, anointing them with oil in the name of the Lord. The prayer of faith will save the sick, and the Lord will raise them up; and anyone who has committed sins will be forgiven. Therefore confess your sins to one another, and pray for one another, so that you may be healed. The prayer of the righteous is powerful and effective. (James 5:14-16, NRSV)

If this ministry is unfamiliar, you may want to locate a church that offers the opportunity for anointing with oil and laying on hands with prayer for healing. Attend. Observe. Ask questions. If your home church already offers this expression of Christ's healing ministry, in what ways could you assist and encourage others to participate?

5. "Jesus Christ is the same yesterday and today and forever" (Heb. 13:8, NRSV). Explore the meaning of this passage for you.

Caring Prayer for Others

God of compassion, source of life and health: strengthen and relieve your servant(s) [*Names (s)*], and give your power of healing to those who minister to their needs, that those for whom our prayers are offered may find help in weakness and have confidence in your loving care; through him who healed the sick and is the physician of our souls, even Jesus Christ our Lord. Amen.[59]

Resting in God's Presence

Now put aside your personal agenda and simply relax, basking in the warmth and healing light of God's love.

Go forth from this special place knowing that the grace and peace of Christ go with you!

AN INVITATION

As I have prayerfully and carefully studied these thirty scripture passages that describe the details and the magnitude of Jesus' healing ministry, a composite picture has emerged. If you have read and meditated on each healing story, you too have been captivated by the consistently caring attitude and inclusive compassion of Jesus. No human need was considered too big or too small for him to address. No health problem was deemed incurable or beyond his help.

Listing all the brokenness and unhealthiness Jesus confronted and cured provides more than sufficient evidence of his personal interest in each individual's salvation, wholeness, and well-being. Consider these health issues that Jesus dealt with during his brief ministry: physical paralysis, blindness, epilepsy, leprosy, dropsy, evil spirits, mental illnesses, hemorrhaging, muteness, deafness, death. Further, Jesus never hesitated to counsel people about their personal relationship with God and with others, knowing that resentment, jealousy, anger, and unforgiveness have a negative impact on one's state of health. Because Jesus cared about the whole person, he intended to help each person he met become whole and healthy in every way possible.

Based on extensive research into the life and ministry of Jesus, coupled with my personal experiences as a committed follower of Jesus, I am convinced that through the Risen Christ, the Holy

Spirit, Jesus is very much alive today and continues to be active throughout the universe and in my personal world. Even as I write these words, my spirit is one with the Spirit of the living Christ. With the ears of my soul and the eyes of my heart I can hear and see the healing Son of God offering you a personal invitation.

An Invitation from Jesus to You, Dear Reader

You are a child of God, created by divine love and grace. Your Creator's greatest desire is not only for you to love your Creator God and to love others as yourself but also for you to be healthy in every area of your life and being. That is why I came many years ago and that is why I come to you this very moment, to give to you hope, help, and health—spiritually, mentally, physically, and in all your relationships. Right now, I invite you to claim and accept for yourself my promises passed on to you by my good friends Matthew, Mark, Luke, and John.

> ❧ "I am the way, and the truth, and the life" (John 14:6, NRSV).

> ❧ "I am the vine, you are the branches. Those who abide in me and I in them bear much fruit, because apart from me you can do nothing" (John 15:5, NRSV).

> ❧ "Ask, and it will be given you; search, and you will find; knock, and the door will be opened for you" (Luke 11:9, NRSV).

> ❧ "Your faith has made you well; go in peace, and be healed of your disease" (Mark 5:34, NRSV).

> ❧ "And remember, I am with you always, to the end of the age" (Matthew 28:20, NRSV).

In the quiet beauty of this sacred moment, I invite you to open your heart, your mind, and your spirit. Trust me confidently, have faith in me completely, allow me to lead you in your next step toward your personal wholeness and health. To help you focus you may want to write down your personal desires and yearnings in these areas of your life:

Spiritual

Mental

Emotional

Physical

Human Relationships

Other Situations

Hold nothing back. Allow me to help you. Bring to me all your cares and worries this day and every day. Right now, call on my strength, forgiveness, grace, and guidance, knowing that I deeply care about you, that I truly understand you, and that I love you unconditionally.

Your Best Friend, Counselor, Redeemer, Healer, and Savior,
Jesus, the Christ

Note to Reader: To accept this personal invitation, pray as your heart connects you with the very heart of God. Get in touch with the spiritual heart of your health and receive new life in Christ. You may want to record thoughts, feelings, directions, instructions, or possible actions. Offer a genuine prayer of thanksgiving for all your blessings and for this special time alone with God. As you move on with your life, go with the assurance that Christ will not let you down and will continue to build you up day by day.

The grace and peace of Christ go with you!

NOTES

1. David Hilton, M.D., "Ethics, World View, and Health," an address to the American Public Health Association, 117th Annual Meeting, October 24, 1989.
2. Howard Clinebell, *Anchoring Your Well Being: Christian Wholeness in a Fractured World* (Nashville, Tenn.: Upper Room Books, 1997), 17.
3. Dale A. Matthews, M.D., *The Faith Factor: Proof of the Healing Power of Prayer* (New York: Viking, 1998), 15–16.
4. Albert E. Day, *Letters on the Healing Ministry* (Nashville, Tenn.: The Upper Room, 1986), 80–81.
5. *The Contemporary English Version* (New York: The American Bible Society, 1995), *v.*
6. Albert E. Day, *Discipline and Discovery* (Springdale, Pa.: Whitaker House, 1988), 11–12.
7. *The Spiritual Formation Bible* (Grand Rapids, Mich.: Zondervan Publishing House, 1999), xv–xvi.
8. These passages from Stephen D. Bryant, foreword to *The Upper Room Disciplines 2000* (Nashville, Tenn.: Upper Room Books, 1999), 11–12.
9. Richard of Chichester, "Three Things We Pray," in *The United Methodist Hymnal* (Nashville, Tenn.: The United Methodist Publishing House, 1989), 493.
10. Day, *Letters on the Healing Ministry*, 7–8.
11. Ibid., 41–42.
12. James W. Moore, *Attitude Is Your Paintbrush: It Colors Every Situation* (Nashville, Tenn.: Dimensions for Living, 1998).
13. Flora Slosson Wuellner, *Prayer, Stress, and Our Inner Wounds* (Nashville, Tenn.: The Upper Room, 1985), 75.
14. For additional discussion of evil, demons, and deliverance ministry see meditations 13, 14, 15.
15. Day, *Letters on the Healing Ministry*, 71.
16. Francis J. Moloney, *Woman, First among the Faithful* (Notre Dame, Ind.: Ave Maria Press, 1986), 18, 20.

17. Elton Trueblood, *Confronting Christ* (Waco, Tex.: Word Books Publisher, 1960), 59–60.

18. René O. Bideux, comp., *A Book of Personal Prayer* (Nashville, Tenn.: Upper Room Books, 1997), 114.

19. Frank Bateman Stanger, *God's Healing Community* (Wilmore, Ky.: Francis Asbury Publishing Company, 1985), 69, 71.

20. Adrian Van Kaam and Susan Muto, *The Power of Appreciation: A New Approach to Personal and Relational Healing* (New York: Crossroads Publishing Company, 1993), 19, 24.

21. Maxie Dunnam, *The Workbook of Intercessory Prayer* (Nashville, Tenn.: The Upper Room, 1979), 91.

22. William Barclay, *The Gospel of Matthew,* rev. ed. The Daily Study Bible Series, vol. 1 (Philadelphia, Pa.: Westminster Press, 1975), 1:304–5.

23. Bideaux, *A Book of Personal Prayer,* 50.

24. Tilda Norberg and Robert D. Webber, *Stretch Out Your Hand: Exploring Healing Prayer* (Nashville, Tenn.: Upper Room Books, 1998), 10.

25. James K. Wagner, *Anna, Jesus Loves You: A Story of Healing and Hope* (Nashville, Tenn.: The Upper Room, 1985), 32.

26. Matthews, *The Faith Factor,* 16.

27. Donald W. Bartow, *The Adventures of Healing,* rev. ed. (Canton, Ohio: Life Enrichment Publishers, 1985), 39.

28. L. David Mitchell, *Liberty in Jesus! Evil Spirits and Exorcism Simply Explained* (Durham, Great Britain: Pentland Press, 1999), 42–43.

29. "The Lord's Prayer," ecumenical text, in *The United Methodist Hymnal,* 894.

30. Francis MacNutt, *Deliverance from Evil Spirits: A Practical Manual* (Grand Rapids, Mich.: Chosen Books, 1995), 46, 32.

31. Day, *Letters on the Healing Ministry,* 42.

32. Michael Perry, "Heal Me, Hands of Jesus," in *The United Methodist Hymnal,* 262.

33. Mildred Thomas, *From Trials to Triumphs* (Dayton, Ohio: UTS Press, 1996), 2–3.

34. G. Ernest Thomas, *Adventurous Living* (Dayton, Ohio: UTS Press, 1998), 9–10.

35. Harvey and Lois Seifert, *Liberation of Life* (Nashville, Tenn.: The Upper Room, 1976), 8.

36. Larry Dossey, M.D., *Healing Words: The Power of Prayer and the Practice of Medicine* (San Francisco: HarperCollins Publishers, 1993), 17–18.

37. Jim Glennon, *Your Healing Is within You* (London: Hodder and Stoughton, 1978), 138.

38. Norberg and Webber, *Stretch Out Your Hand,* 73–74.

39. Francis MacNutt, *The Power to Heal* (Notre Dame, Ind.: Ave Maria Press, 1977), 62.

40. Elton Trueblood, as quoted in James K. Wagner, *An Adventure in Healing and Wholeness: The Healing Ministry of Christ in the World Today* (Nashville, Tenn.: Upper Room Books, l993), 74.

41. Catherine Marshall, *Something More: In Search of a Deeper Faith* (New York: Avon Books, l974), 144–45.

42. Steve Harper, *Praying through the Lord's Prayer* (Nashville, Tenn.: Upper Room Books, l992), 96–97.

43. Clara H. Scott, "Open My Eyes, That I May See," in *The United Methodist Hymnal*, 454.

44. Albert Schweitzer, *The Quest of the Historical Jesus* (New York: Macmillan, 1959), 401.

45. *The United Methodist Hymnal*, 454, 359, 378.

46. Rueben P. Job and Norman Shawchuck, *A Guide to Prayer for All God's People* (Nashville, Tenn.: Upper Room Books, 1990), 153.

47. From Preface of Christian Death 1, *The Roman Missal: The Sacramentary* (Collegeville, Minn.: The Liturgical Press, 1974), 493.

48. James K. Wagner, *Blessed to Be a Blessing: How to Have an Intentional Healing Ministry in Your Church* (Nashville, Tenn.: The Upper Room, 1980), 73.

49. Tommy Tyson, quoted in Wagner, *An Adventure in Healing and Wholeness*, 55.

50. Anne S. White, *Healing Devotions: Daily Meditations and Prayers Based on Scriptures and Hymns* (New York: Morehouse-Barlow Co., l975), 121.

51. Laurence Hull Stookey, "For Those Who Mourn," in *The United Methodist Hymnal*, 461.

52. From Introduction to "Healing Services and Prayers," in *The United Methodist Book of Worship* (Nashville, Tenn.: The United Methodist Publishing House, l992), 613–14.

53. Trueblood, *Confronting Christ*, 57.

54. Francis MacNutt, quoted in *United Methodist Reporter* (Dallas, Tex., 17 August, 1979).

55. Donald Bartow, *The Healing Service* (Canton, Ohio: Life Enrichment Publishers, 1974), 15.

56. Norberg and Webber, *Stretch Out Your Hand*, 32.

57. Wagner, *An Adventure in Healing and Wholeness*, 32.

58. Day, *Letters on the Healing Ministry*, 130.

59. Laurence Hull Stookey, "For the Sick" (alt.) in *The United Methodist Hymnal*, 457.

RESOURCES

Bartow, Donald W. *The Adventures of Healing*. Rev. ed. Canton, Ohio: Life Enrichment Publishers, 1985.

Clinebell, Howard. *Anchoring Your Well Being: Christian Wholeness in a Fractured World*. Nashville, Tenn.: Upper Room Books, 1997.

Day, Albert E. *Discipline and Discovery*. Rev. ed. Nashville, Tenn.: The Disciplined Order of Christ, 1988.

———. *Letters on the Healing Ministry*. Nashville, Tenn.: The Upper Room, 1990. (These titles by Day are available by contacting: Disciplined Order of Christ, P.O. Box 753, Ashland, OH 44805–4529, Phone and FAX 1-419–281–3932.)

DelBene, Ron, Herb Montgomery and Mary Montgomery. *The Breath of Life: A Workbook*. Nashville, Tenn.: Upper Room Books, 1996.

Donnelly, Doris. *Learning to Forgive*. Nashville, Tenn.: Abingdon Press, 1986.

Dossey, Larry, M.D. *Healing Words: The Power of Prayer and the Practice of Medicine*. San Francisco, Calif.: HarperSanFrancisco, 1993.

Dunnam, Maxie. *The Workbook of Intercessory Prayer*. Nashville, Tenn.: The Upper Room, 1979.

———. *The Workbook of Living Prayer*. Nashville, Tenn.: The Upper Room, 1974.

Foster, Richard J. *Prayer: Finding the Heart's True Home*. San Francisco, Calif.: HarperSanFrancisco, 1992.

Job, Rueben P. and Norman Shawchuck. *A Guide to Prayer for Ministers and Other Servants*. Nashville, Tenn.: The Upper Room, 1983.

———. *A Guide to Prayer for All God's People*. Nashville, Tenn.: Upper Room Books, 1990.

MacNutt, Francis. *Deliverance from Evil Spirits: A Practical Manual*. Grand Rapids, Mich.: Chosen Books, 1995.

Matthews, Dale A. *The Faith Factor: Proof of the Healing Power of Prayer*. New York: Viking, 1998.

Mitchell, L. David. *Liberty in Jesus! Evil Spirits and Exorcism Simply Explained*. Durham, Great Britain: Pentland Press, 1999.

Morris, Danny E. *Yearning to Know God's Will: A Workbook for Discerning God's Guidance for Your Life*. Grand Rapids, Mich.: Zondervan, 1991.

Mulholland, M. Robert, Jr., *Shaped by the Word: The Power of Scripture in Spiritual Formation*. Rev. ed. Nashville, Tenn.: Upper Room Books, 2000.

Norberg, Tilda and Robert D. Webber. *Stretch Out Your Hand: Exploring Healing Prayer*. Nashville, Tenn.: Upper Room Books, 1998.

Pearson, Mark A. *Christian Healing: A Practical and Comprehensive Guide*. 2nd ed. Grand Rapids, Mich.: Chosen Books, 1995.

Smedes, Lewis B. *The Art of Forgiving*. New York: Ballantine, 1996.

Stanger, Frank Bateman. *God's Healing Community*. Wilmore, Ky.: Francis Asbury Publishing, 1985.

Van Kaam, Adrian and Susan Muto. *The Power of Appreciation: A New Approach to Personal and Relational Healing*. New York: Crossroads, 1993.

Wagner, James K. *An Adventure in Healing and Wholeness: The Healing Ministry of Christ in the Church Today*. Nashville, Tenn.: Upper Room Books, 1993.

———. *Blessed to Be a Blessing: How to Have an Intentional Healing Ministry in Your Church*. Nashville, Tenn.: The Upper Room, 1980.

Weatherhead, Leslie. *The Will of God* (Workbook Edition by Rebecca Laird). Nashville, Tenn.: Abingdon Press, 1995.

Wuellner, Flora S. *Feed My Shepherds: Spiritual Healing and Renewal for Those in Christian Leadership*. Nashville, Tenn.: Upper Room Books, 1998.

———. *Forgiveness, the Passionate Journey: Nine Steps of Forgiving through Jesus' Beatitudes*. Nashville, Tenn.: Upper Room Books, 2001.

———. *Prayer, Stress, and Our Inner Wounds*. Nashville, Tenn.: The Upper Room, 1985.

———. *Prayer and Our Bodies*. Nashville, Tenn.: The Upper Room, 1987.

———. *Release: Healing from Wounds of Family, Church, and Community*. Nashville, Tenn.: Upper Room Books, 1996.

For a listing of spiritual-formation resources published by Upper Room Ministries, visit http://www.upperroom.org.

SCRIPTURE INDEX*

INDIVIDUAL HEALINGS BY JESUS

	Matthew	Mark	Luke	John
1. Nobleman's son				4:46-53
2. Uncle's spirit		1:21-28	4:31-37	
3. Simon's mother-in-law	8:14-15	1:29-31	4:38-39	
4. A leper	8:1-4	1:40-45	5:12-16	
5. Paralytic carried by four	9:1-8	2:1-12	5:17-26	
6. Sick man at the pool				5:1-15
7. Withered hand	12:9-14	3:1-6	6:6-11	
8. Centurion's servant	8:5-13		7:2-10	
9. Widow's son raised			7:11-17	
10. Demoniac(s) at Gadara	8:28-34	5:1-20	8:26-36	
11. Issue of blood	9:20-22	5:25-34	8:43-48	
12. Jairus's daughter raised	9:18-26	5:21-43	8:40-56	
13. Two blind men	9:27-31			
14. Dumb devil possessed	9:32-34			
15. Daughter of Canaan woman	15:21-28	7:24-30		
16. Deaf, speech impediment		7:32-37		
17. Blind man of Bethsaida		8:22-26		
18. Epileptic boy	17:14-21	9:14-29	9:37-42	
19. Man born blind				9:1-41
20. Man blind, mute, possessed	12:22-28		11:14-23	
21. Women bent over			13:10-17	
22. Man with dropsy			14:1-5	
23. Raising of Lazarus				11:1-44
24. Ten lepers			17:11-19	
25. Blind Bartimaeus		10:46-52	18:35-43	
26. Two blind men	20:29-34			

* James K. Wagner, comp., study guide to *Letters on the Healing Ministry,* by Albert E. Day (Nashville, Tenn.: The Upper Room, 1964), 116–18.

MULTIPLE HEALINGS BY JESUS

	Matthew	Mark	Luke	Acts
1. Crowd at Peter's door	8:16-17	1:32-34	4:40-41	
2. Crowds after leper healed			5:15-16	
3. Crowd near Capernaum	12:15-21	3:7-12		
4. Answering John's question	11:2-6		7:18-23	
5. Before feeding the 5,000	14:13-14		9:11	
6. At Gennesaret	14:34-36	6:53-56		
7. Before feeding 4,000	15:29-31			
8. Crowds beyond the Jordan	19:1-2			
9. Blind & lame in temple	21:14			
10. Some sick in Nazareth	13:54-58	6:1-6		
11. All kinds of sickness	4:23-24	6:56		
12. Every sickness & disease	9:35			
13. All oppressed				10:38

INDIVIDUAL HEALINGS BY THE APOSTLES

	Acts
1. The man lame from birth	3:1-10
2. Paul regains his sight	9:1-19; 22:1-13
3. Aeneas the paralytic	9:32-35
4. Raising of Dorcas	9:36-42
5. Crippled man by Lystra	14:8-18
6. Girl with a spirit of divination	16:16-18
7. Eutychus restored to life	20:7-12
8. Paul healed of snakebite	28:1-6
9. Father of Publius healed	28:7-8

MULTIPLE HEALINGS BY THE APOSTLES

	Acts
1. Many wonders and signs	2:43
2. Many sick healed in Jerusalem	5:12-16
3. Stephen performs many miracles	6:8
4. Philip heals many at Samaria	8:5-13
5. Paul and Barnabas work signs and wonders	14:3
6. Paul heals at Ephesus	19:11-12
7. Sick healed at Melita	28:9

SOME OTHER NEW TESTAMENT SCRIPTURES

1. Instructions of Jesus and
   promises to believers   Mark 16:14-20; Luke 10:8-9
2. Signs and wonders   Rom. 15:18-19
        2 Cor. 12:12; Heb. 2:4
3. Healing   1 Cor. 12:9; 12:28-30
4. Anointing   Mark 6:13; James 5:14
5. Perfect eternal healing   Rev. 21:1-6

SOME OLD TESTAMENT REFERENCES TO HEALING

1. None of these diseases   Exod. 15:26
2. The fiery serpent   Num. 21:6-9
3. Shunammite's son raised   2 Kings 4:18-37
4. Naaman healed   2 Kings 5:1-14
5. Hezekiah healed   2 Kings 20:1-11
6. "With his stripes we are healed" (KJV)   Isa. 53:5
7. Some healing psalms   Pss. 23; 30; 103
8. Dead man raised   2 Kings 13:20-21

ABOUT THE AUTHOR

James K. Wagner is a writer and the former Director of Prayer and Healing Ministries at The Upper Room in Nashville, Tennessee. Dr. Wagner holds a Doctor of Ministry degree in the area of the Healing Ministry of the Church as well as the Master of Divinity degree, both from United Theological Seminary in Dayton, Ohio. Now retired, Dr. Wagner was a United Methodist minister for thirty-one years, serving churches in Ohio. He also served as executive director of The Disciplined Order of Christ and continues an active role in that organization.

ACKNOWLEDGMENTS

The English translation of the Preface for the Mass of the Dead from *The Roman Missal* © 1973, International Committee on English in the Liturgy, Inc. All rights reserved.

Excerpts from *Letters on the Healing Ministry* by Albert E. Day. Copyright © 1990 by The Disciplined Order of Christ, 1155 S. Columbus St., Ashland, Ohio 44805-4529.

"The Lord's Prayer" ecumenical text. Used by permission of the International Consultation on English Texts.

Excerpts from "Heal Me, Hands of Jesus" verses 1 and 4 by Michael Perry. Copyright © 1982 Hope Publishing Co., Carol Stream, IL 60188. All rights reserved. Used by permission.

"The Scriptures and Healing." Used by permission of The Total Living Center, Canton, Ohio.

"For Those Who Mourn" by Laurence Hull Stookey from *The United Methodist Hymnal.* Copyright © 1989 The United Methodist Publishing House. Used by permission.

"For the Sick" from *The Book of Common Prayer,* alt. by Laurence Hull Stookey. Alt. © 1989 The United Methodist Publishing House. Used by permission.